THE HUMAN HEART

A CONSUMER'S GUIDE TO CARDIAC CARE

THE HUMAN HEART

A CONSUMER'S GUIDE TO CARDIAC CARE

BRENDAN PHIBBS, M.D., F.A.C.P., F.A.C.C.

Chief of Medicine and Director of Cardiology,
Kino Community Hospital,
Tucson, Arizona;
Clinical Professor of Medicine, Section of Cardiology,
University of Arizona Medical School,
Tucson, Arizona

with 154 illustrations

A PLUME BOOK

NEW AMERICAN LIBRARY

MOSBY

TIMES MIRROR
NEW YORK AND SCARBOROUGH, ONTARIO

Publisher: Thomas A. Manning
Assistant editor: Nancy L. Mullins
Manuscript editor: Kathy Brown
Production: Margaret B. Bridenbaugh

MOSBY MEDICAL LIBRARY

This is a revised edition of a book previously published
by The C.V. Mosby Company entitled
THE HUMAN HEART:
A GUIDE TO HEART DISEASE.

NAL books are available at quantity discounts
when used to promote products or services. For information
please write to Premium Marketing Division,
The New American Library, Inc.,
1633 Broadway, New York, New York 10019.

PLUME TRADEMARK REG. U.S. PAT. OFF. AND FOREIGN COUNTRIES
REGISTERED TRADEMARK—MARCA REGISTRADA
HECHO EN FORGE VILLAGE, MASS., U.S.A.

SIGNET, SIGNET CLASSICS, MENTOR, PLUME, MERIDIAN and
NAL BOOKS are published by The New American Library, Inc.,
1633 Broadway, New York, New York 10019, in Canada, by
The New American Library of Canada, Limited,
81 Mack Avenue, Scarborough, Ontario M1L 1M8.

Library of Congress Cataloging in Publication Data
Phibbs, Brendan.
The human heart.
"A Plume book."
Bibliography: p.
1. Heart—Diseases. 2. Cardiology—Popular
works. I. Title.
RC681.P53 1982 616.1'2 82-2119
ISBN 0-452-25337-3 AACR2

1 2 3 4 5 6 7 8 9 02/A/234
Printed in the United States of America

To the memory of my wife
Penny
who contended with medical school,
the army camps and separation of war,
four children, my sometimes unforgiveable disposition,
the blizzards of Wyoming, and the sandstorms of Arizona,

with love and gratitude

Preface

Twenty years ago a cardiologist was likely to be a thoughtful physician who listened to your symptoms, carried out a particularly careful physical examination, recorded an electrocardiogram, made an x-ray examination of your chest, and told you what he thought was wrong with you. Within the limits of human fallibility, you could usually believe him. You could also rely on his advice when he recommended treatment or further evaluation. There was no reason, economic or otherwise, for him to tell you anything but the truth as nearly as he could determine it.

The earlier editions of this book were written to help patients cooperate with that kind of physician in the diagnosis and treatment of their heart disease. Any cardiac patient should understand the basic structure and function of the heart; the patient should understand what heart disease is present, how the diagnosis was reached, and what the characteristics of the disease are; finally, the patient should understand thoroughly the benefits and hazards of the treatment recommended as well as the ultimate outlook in terms of longevity and function. Given the same risks, an informed patient will always fare better and live longer than an uninformed one. This kind of education of patients about their disease and its significance is one purpose of this book and a very important one.

Times change, not always for the better.

This new edition is written with a second purpose, to meet an immediate and frightening need.

The past two decades have seen an explosion of high-technology cardiology. It is now possible to insert catheters and recording instruments inside the chambers of the heart to detect and to measure disease of the valves, the coronary arteries, and the heart muscle itself with incredible accuracy.

Twenty years ago there was nothing much anyone could do about heart block in its more serious forms; sooner or later patients with heart block simply died. Now, thanks to electronic pacemakers, these patients can often be guaranteed years of productive life.

Diseased heart valves that would have led to invalidism and death twenty years ago can now be replaced. Coronary arteries that are blocked with masses of fat can be bypassed with new vessels, creating a "detour" around the obstruction. These are real miracles of modern science and uncounted thousands owe their health and their very lives to them.

Now for the other side of the coin.

The national bill for just one type of cardiac catheterization—coronary arteriography—is about 500 million dollars per year. The annual cost for one kind of heart surgery—coronary artery bypass grafting—is well into the billions. It is common for cardiologists and cardiac surgeons to generate six and seven figure annual incomes performing these procedures. To paraphrase Lord Acton, "Enormous profits corrupt enormously." *In recent years it has become painfully clear that many of these expensive and often dangerous procedures are being performed when there is no justification for them.*

What are the dimensions of the problem? A number of responsible cardiologists have estimated that as many as half the cardiac catheterizations carried out to detect coronary disease in the United States today are not justified by any reasonable medical criteria.

Coronary artery bypass surgery is by far the commonest form of heart surgery in the United States today. The risk of dying of the procedure ranges from 2% to 10%. It would be conservative to state that a third of all coronary artery bypass graft procedures carried out in the United States each year are not justified by any available scientific data; a more accurate figure might be something like 50%.

The insertion of pacemakers may represent the most flagrant problem of all. In the August 14, 1981, issue of the *Journal of the American Medical Association* a group of cardiologists from Brooklyn reported their experience in evaluating the need for pacemaker insertion in a number of cases. These cardiologists associated with Downstate Medical School of New York set up reasonable criteria to establish which pacemaker insertions were justified and which were not. When these criteria were put into effect, *the number of pacemaker insertions fell by 70% over a two-year period.* In other words presumably only about 30% of the pacemakers previously being inserted were needed.

In short, there has been a frightening metamorphosis in recent years so that all too often the patient is not a victim of heart disease but rather of the medical profession or at least of a small segment of it.

When members of the public learn of this kind of abuse and exploitation, they are properly outraged, and they demand that something be done about it. The leaders of American cardiology are in complete agreement; abuse exists and "something should be done about it," but precisely *what* is the question. Trying to bring a runaway multibillion dollar industry under control is slow and sometimes hazardous; some wit commented that for every unscrupulous physician there are two unscrupulous lawyers ready to take his side.

Standards are slowly being promulgated, and review mechanisms are being organized, but the process is slow and often cumbersome. A more direct approach is needed, and this approach in the view of a number of prominent cardiologists is *education of the public.* The cardiac patient today needs a guide through the jungle of profitable technology to avoid exploitation or even to survive.

This book therefore has been rewritten to give the cardiac patient the information needed to participate intelligently in decisions about diagnosis and treatment and to question those decisions when they seem inappropriate.

In the first part of the book the structure and function of the heart are described in health and in disease. Such common questions as "What is heart failure?" and "Where are the coronary arteries?" are answered. In subsequent sections the major specific diseases affecting the heart are described in detail. After reading each section the patient should be able to make reasonable decisions about appropriate diagnostic procedures and treatment for that kind of disease.

There is a question section after many of the major chapters; these questions suggest the items of information that the patient should have acquired or at times the questions that the patient should ask the cardiologist when certain procedures are recommended.

When coronary arteriography is recommended, for example, the cardiac patient should know what the coronary arteries are and how they function; terms like "coronary atheromatosis," "angina pectoris," "myocardial infarction," "left-main disease," or "three-vessel disease" should be familiar and should be thoroughly understood. This will involve no more than a few hours' reading; after all there are only three coronary arteries!

Before submitting to coronary artery bypass graft surgery the patient should understand exactly what the procedure is and what the risks are. The patient should also understand the purpose of the surgery, that is, whether the surgery is being proposed simply to relieve cardiac pain or if it is hoped that it will prolong the patient's life and, if so, whether this is a reasonable hope given the type of disease present.

The patient confronted with pacemaker insertion should understand the structure and function of the electric system that originates and conducts the heartbeat. This is a surprisingly simple system with only five basic elements; learning about it is not a formidable assignment. Before submitting to pacemaker insertion for a sick sinus syndrome the patient should know what the sinus node is and what criteria are needed to establish the diagnosis of subnormal sinus node function. The patient with atrioventricular (AV) block should understand the difference between AV nodal block and bundle-branch block; Wenckebach block and Mobitz type II block should be thoroughly distinguished in the patient's mind. To understand all this the patient should know what these types of block look like on an electrocardiogram; again, this is surprisingly easy to do. As I like to tell my medical students, one who can count simple numbers from three to five and distinguish up from down can diagnose the major types of heart block.

In its second purpose this book is an attempt to do something that has never been done before, that is, to present the cardiac patient with enough specific technical information to permit intelligent participation in decisions about diagnosis and treatment and to present that information in terms sufficiently clear and simple that the patient can comprehend it with a few hours' reading.

There has never been any question that accurate, relevant medical information helps patients deal with any disease; in today's world the cardiac patient must take a giant stride in level of medical education and become an active participant rather than a passive object. The patient's very survival may be at stake.

I hope this book may have some small influence in bringing a degree of openness and honesty to the relations of patients with physicians; possibly that openness may redirect some part of the medical profession toward those ideals of dedication, unselfishness, and high purpose that sustained our greatest healers.

For the sake of simplicity and clarity, the term "he" will be used to refer to the physician, although I am well aware many cardiologists and cardiac surgeons are women.   **Brendan Phibbs, M.D.**

Contents

1   Structure of the heart

The structure of the heart is surprisingly simple; a half hour's easy reading will give you all the information you need for practical purposes. It consists of (1) four heart chambers, (2) four heart valves, (3) four layers of the heart wall, (4) six great vessels leading the blood into and out of the chambers of the heart, and (5) three coronary arteries.

THE CHAMBERS OF THE HEART

The heart is a hollow organ made up of four chambers, two above and two below. The two top chambers are called the "atria"; the term comes from a Latin word meaning "anteroom" or porch. These are small, thin-walled structures that act chiefly as reservoirs for the blood returning to the heart from the veins; in function they are like porches or entryways to the powerful chambers below.

The ventricles are large, thick-walled chambers that do the real work of pumping the blood. ("Ventriculus," the Latin word for cavity or pouch, is the origin of this term.) These chambers form the great mass of the heart.

Look at Fig. 1-1. Notice the wall or septum that divides the right atrium from the left atrium and the right ventricle from the left ventricle. In other words, the right atrium and right ventricle together form the right side of the heart, and the left atrium and left ventricle together form the left side. The wall of tissue that divides the heart into left and right halves is much like the septum that divides your nose into right and left nostrils. The important thing to remember about this septum is that it is absolutely watertight or more properly, bloodtight. Normally no blood can pass through this septum from one side of the heart to the other. (It took the human race about 4,000 years to discover this fact. The ancient Greeks and Romans were convinced that blood must somehow ooze through the septum from one side of the heart to the other. It doesn't.)

Physicians commonly refer to the right atrium and right ventricle together as the **right heart** and the left atrium and left ventricle together as the **left heart.** (Your physician may use the word **"auricle"** instead of atrium. This is somewhat older usage common in the United States.)

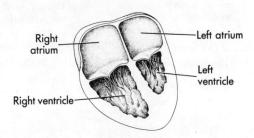

Fig. 1-1. Chambers of the heart.

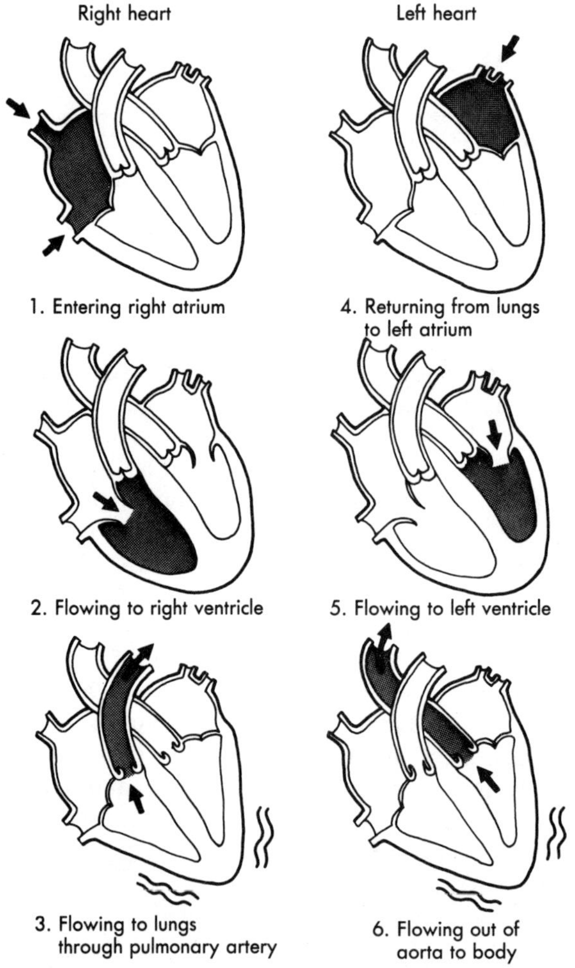

Fig. 1-2. Connections of the heart and lungs. Movement of the blood into the right heart, from the right heart to the lungs, from the lungs to the left heart, and on to the blood vessels of the body.

CONNECTIONS OF THE HEART AND LUNGS

The cardiac septum is a watertight barrier. Nothing can move through it from the right side of the heart to the left side. That observation worried the human race for thousands of years; if the blood cannot move through the septum, how does it ever move forward; that is, how does it circulate? Why doesn't it bring up short against the septum like water against a dam? Many ingenious theories were proposed, but they were all wrong; it wasn't until the seventeenth century that the great Englishman, William Harvey, discovered a titanic truth. There are no normal direct connections between the right heart and the left heart; the blood must move from the right heart to the left heart by way of the lungs.

The heart is thus a double pump; the right heart pulls the blood out of the veins and pumps it into the lungs; the left heart pulls the blood out of the lungs and pumps it on to the body (Fig. 1-2).

GREAT VESSELS OF THE HEART

The great vessels of the heart (Fig. 1-3) is the term used to describe the arteries and veins attached to the heart. They are as follows:

1. The top and bottom **venae cavae** or cavernous veins—huge structures that carry the blood from all over the body back to the top and bottom of the right atrium respectively.
2. The **pulmonary artery**—the outlet of the right ventricle. It branches out into the lungs like a profuse tree.
3. The **pulmonary veins**—the vessels that carry the oxygenated blood back from the lungs to the left atrium.
4. The **aorta** or great artery—carries the oxygenated blood out of the left ventricle to the body.

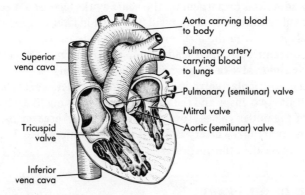

Fig. 1-3. The great arteries and veins connecting with the heart. The superior and inferior venae cavae carry blood from the body to the right heart; the pulmonary artery carries the blood to the lungs; the pulmonary veins (not shown here and actually behind the aorta) return the blood to the left heart and the aorta carries the oxygenated blood on out to the body.

VALVES OF THE HEART

Like any pump, the heart has valves to keep the blood flowing in the right direction. Proper function of these small flaps of tissue spells the difference between health and sickness or life and death.

Almost everyone is familiar with the word "valve." Very few people really know what a valve is or what it does. Imagine pumping water through a pipe with an old-fashioned farm pump. To keep the water from flowing back toward the pump between strokes, one could place a valve in the pipe leading out of the pump. The simplest kind of valve would consist of two semicircular flaps hinged to open only one way, forward with the flow of water. These flaps would close the pipe completely when they swung shut. When the water flowed forward from the pump, the flaps of the valve would swing open, allowing the water to pass. Between strokes the valves would snap shut if any water attempted to flow back toward the pump (Fig. 1-4).

The heart is equipped with four sets of valves that function on this simple principle.

A valve is located between each atrium and ventricle (Fig. 1-5). These valves open downward into the ventricle. When the atria contract, the valves swing open, allowing the blood to flow down into the ventricles. When the ventricles contract, these valves snap shut, preventing any blood from flowing back up into the atria.

A valve is also located at the outlet from each ventricle into the great vessel leaving the chamber. When the ventricles contract, these valves are forced open; the blood rushes into the pulmonary artery and the aorta. When the ventricles relax, the valves close, shutting off any backward flow into the ventricles.

If the heart is to function efficiently, these valves must be absolutely watertight. Furthermore, they must open freely and widely to let the blood flow forward with the pumping action of the heart. If the valves leak or if they are held partly shut by adhesions or hardening, the heart works against a mechanical load, often an impossible and fatal load, as will be shown in later chapters.

The valves between the atria and ventricles are called the **atrioventricular valves.** The atrioventricular valve leading into the right ventricle has three flaps: it is called the **tricuspid valve** (a cusp is a valve flap or leaflet).

The atrioventricular valve that swings into the left ventricle is called the **mitral valve.** It has two cusps and therefore looks something like a bishop's mitre.

Each of the outlet valves from the ventricles has three cusps. The valve at the entry to the pulmonary artery is called the **pulmonic valve.** The valve at the entry to the aorta is called the **aortic valve.**

LAYERS OF THE HEART

The heart does not simply hang freely in the chest cavity; around it is a loose protective sack of tissue called the **pericardium.** The heart lies inside this sack, which is loose enough to permit the heart to beat easily. Picture a turnip

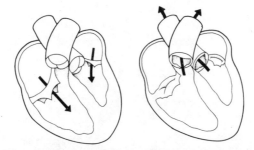

Fig. 1-4. The inlet and outlet valves of the ventricles. The two atrioventricular valves (left side) open to let the blood flow from atria to ventricles. Semilunar valves at the beginning of the two great arteries swing open to let the blood leave the ventricles, from right ventricle to lungs and from left ventricle to the body.

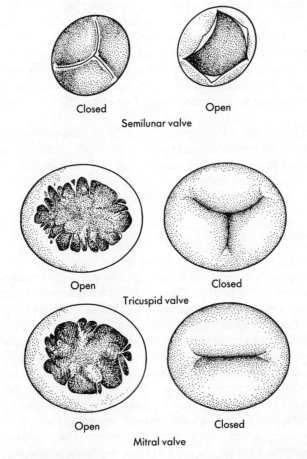

Closed   Open
             Semilunar valve

Open   Closed
             Tricuspid valve

Open   Closed
              Mitral valve

Fig. 1-5. Valves of the heart viewed from above as they open and close.

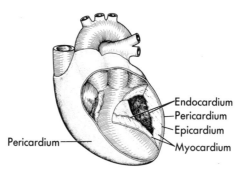

Fig. 1-6. Layers of the heart.

held in a heavy, double-thickness plastic bag. This is about the way the heart looks inside the pericardium (Fig. 1-6).

If the pericardium is cut open, the surface of the heart itself appears shiny and reddish. One can actually peel away a thin, shiny membrane from the surface of the heart. This membrane is called the **epicardium** (Fig. 1-6).

The mass of the heart muscle; under the epicardium is a thick layer of muscle called the **myocardium,** which forms the actual working part of the heart. The myocardium is thickest in the left ventricle; it is thinnest in the atria. The cells in the myocardium are a specialized kind of muscle, different from anything else in the body.

The inside of the heart, or cavity, is lined with another smooth, shiny membrane much like the inside surface of one's cheek. This thin, smooth, shiny membrane covers the inside of the chambers of the heart; it also covers the heart valves and the small muscles associated with the opening and closing of these valves. This is called the **endocardium** (Fig. 1-6).

BLOOD SUPPLY OF THE HEART

It seems odd that the tissues making up the heart must have their own separate blood supply. One might think that the torrent of blood rushing through the heart every minute would be more than adequate for the needs of the organ itself. The walls of the heart, however, consist of layers of muscle of a particular specialized type. These walls are quite thick—the wall of the left ventricle is often over 1 inch thick. Since the lining of the heart is watertight, the blood cannot seep out through the layers of muscle to provide the nourishment essential to these constantly working masses of muscle. Blood is carried through the muscle layers that form the wall of the heart by means of the two **coronary arteries.** These small vessels branch off the aorta just after it leaves the heart and curl back across the surface of the chambers, sending twigs through the walls (Fig. 1-7).

The coronary arteries are so named because of the supposed resemblance to a crown or ''corona'' of the little arteries as they encircle the heart. These arteries divide into smaller and smaller branches like all blood vessels in the body,

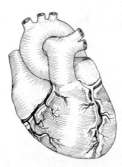

Fig. 1-7. The coronary arteries and veins. These vessels course across the surface of the heart sending branches down into the muscle and throughout the inner structure of the heart.

until they become so small that only one blood cell at a time can move through them. At this point the vessels are called **capillaries.** After the blood has passed through the capillaries and the tissues have extracted the needed oxygen from it, it returns by way of veins, which become larger and larger until they, like all other veins in the body, empty into the right atrium. The veins from the wall of the heart, or coronary veins, empty into the right atrium through a structure called the **coronary sinus.**

The blood supply of the tissues in the wall of the heart is not very good; thousands of people die every year because of this curious fact. In most organs and tissues of the body there is a "reserve" or collateral blood supply. In each finger, for instance, there are two arteries, one on each side. These arteries are connected by many cross-channels, or collateral vessels. If the artery is cut on one side, the collateral or cross-connections from the artery on the other would probably provide sufficient blood to maintain life in the tissues of the finger. The same "safety" feature is true in most of the major areas of the body. It is **not** true in the wall of the heart.

The coronary arteries are **end arteries,** meaning that each branch follows its own course to some area of the heart muscle with relatively few connections with other branches nearby. If one of these coronary branches is stopped up by hardening or by a blood clot, the muscle that depends on it for blood will die. A form of gangrene actually sets in. (Some people's coronary arteries have many more cross-connections than others. The more of these cross-connections, or collateral vessels, an individual has the less likely he is to die of coronary artery disease. In 10,000 or 20,000 years the process of evolution may result in a race with a good coronary blood supply by virtue of the early death of those without it.)

2   Function of the heart

Blood is pumped through the chambers of the heart and out through the great vessels by a simple squeezing action of the heart chambers (Fig. 2-1). You have probably seen a bulb syringe with a glass nozzle. Suppose it to be full of water. If you squeezed forcefully, expelling the water, you would be imitating the contraction of a heart chamber. This is called **systole** (sis-toe-lee). After the syringe had been emptied, imagine that you placed the nozzle in a container of water and let the bulb expand so that it filled. This is what a heart chamber does when it relaxes and fills with blood. The movement is called **diastole** (die-as-toe-lee).

One can picture the whole process by holding the left hand over the right, fists clenched. If the left hand represents the atria, the right hand will represent the ventricles. Now clench the left fist—the atria—while opening the right fist—the ventricles. This is what happens during atrial systole when the atria are pumping blood down into the ventricles. Next, open the left fist and clench the right. This is what happens during ventricular systole when the ventricles are pumping blood out into the two great arteries and the atria are refilling. By alternately opening and clenching the two fists you can form a good idea of the coordinated beat of the heart.

The whole cycle of a heartbeat, in other words, goes through these stages:

1. **Atrial systole:** The atria contract, forcing the blood down into the ventricles.
2. **Ventricular systole:** The ventricles contract, forcing the blood out the pulmonary artery and aorta.
3. **Atrial diastole:** This starts during ventricular systole as the atria begin refilling with blood from the great veins.
4. **Ventricular diastole:** This takes place during atrial systole as blood from the atria fills the ventricles.

ELECTRIC CONTROL OF THE HEARTBEAT

Like the engine in your car the heart depends on electrical energy to start it and keep it going. Specifically the heart beats because a wave of electricity moves through the tissues of the chambers, starting in the atria and moving down to the ventricles. This electric wave makes the muscle wall of each chamber contract, pumping out its contained blood.

Most of the muscles in the body depend on a nerve connection to the brain for the electric activation that starts their movement. If the nerves connecting the brain to the muscles of the arm, for example, are cut anywhere along the course, the arm will be paralyzed. The heart is different because it has its own electrical circuit and "spark plug"; it needs no connection to the rest of the nervous system (Fig. 2-2).

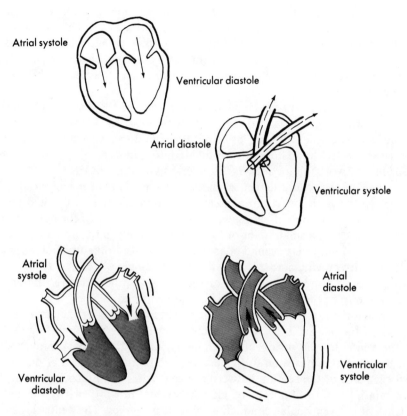

Fig. 2-1. Systole and diastole. Systole means contraction or squeezing together. Diastole means expansion and refilling.

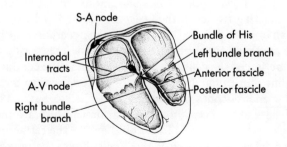

Fig. 2-2. The pacemaking and conducting tissues of the heart—the tissues that generate the electric impulse that activates the heartbeat and that conduct it through the chambers. For explanation and diagram of ECG waves, see Fig. 4-1.

The electric wave that starts the heartbeat comes from a tiny bundle of nerve tissue in the right atrium called the **sinoatrial node.** This is the normal pacemaker of the heart. From this bit of nerve tissue an electric wave starts out across the atria, spreading through the muscle like a ripple across a pond. In the wake of this wave of electric energy the atria contracts, forcing the blood down into the ventricles.

The next structure in the conducting system of the heart is a connecting "nerve" between the atria and the ventricles called the **atrioventricular node.** This node soon divides into two branches that run down each side of the septum between the ventricles. These in turn divide into hundreds of tiny nerve fibrils, ending in a network that permeates the muscle walls of the heart.

Imagine that you, the reader, suddenly have a kind of magic eyesight; you can see electricity the way you can see light. Imagine that you could actually watch the spread of this activating wave through the tissues of the heart. You see the sinoatrial node, a small point of light, glowing dully in the upper right corner of the right atrium. Every second or so this point winks brilliantly and sends a rim of glowing fire moving across the atria. This is a single wave, like a single ripple moving across a pond. As this wave of energy passes, the atria are stimulated to contract, pumping their load of blood into the ventricles.

When the expanding ring of light reaches the edges of the atria, it winks out, except for one small spark that moves down the nerve connecting the atria and the ventricle, the atrioventricular node. At first the spark moves slowly through this nerve, but soon it divides into two points of light that dart swiftly down each side of the septum between the ventricles. With dazzling speed, each spark multiplies into hundreds of glowing points, moving swiftly through the branches of the ventricular conducting system, or nerves. The ventricles sparkle like a suddenly illuminated Christmas tree, and then as suddenly fall dark. The muscular walls are stung into action, and the life-giving flood of blood pours out of each ventricle.

By this simple electric system the beat of the chambers is coordinated. The ventricles contract when they are at their peak distention, filled to capacity with blood. This makes for maximum efficiency and heart performance. If the ventricles contracted when they were only half filled, for example, the heart would have to beat about twice as fast to pump the same amount of blood per minute.

The conducting tissues in the heart are formed of living cells. Each time they transmit an impulse they are fatigued; it takes a certain time before they have recovered and are ready for their next transmission. This period of time is called the **refractory period** of the cells. Picture the tissues in the conducting network of the heart as a line of men handing heavy stones along, one to the next. Each man can pass only so many stones per minute. After he has handed one stone to his next worker, it takes him a certain amount of time to turn around and reach out his arms to pick up the next one. This would be like the refractory period of the heart cells. The refractory period of these cells limits the number of times per minute that the heart can beat. It is the reason, for instance, that the heart cannot beat 500 times a minute since the conducting tissues cannot perform that many transmissions any more than a man could pass a heavy stone to his fellow 500

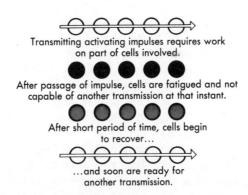

Transmitting activating impulses requires work
on part of cells involved.

After passage of impulse, cells are fatigued and not
capable of another transmission at that instant.

After short period of time, cells begin
to recover...

...and soon are ready for
another transmission.

Fig. 2-3. Refractory period. Fatigue and recovery of conducting cells.

times a minute. In some abnormal states the heart may actually beat over 300 times a minute, but this cannot be kept up indefinitely.

The rhythm of the heartbeat is usually regular. Under normal conditions, however, it may change. Fear or anger will often speed the heart, and overactivity of certain nerves may slow it. These changes occur because the heart is to some extent under the control of nerves connected to the brain. There are two major types of nerves traveling to the conducting tissues in the atria and in the atrioventricular node. One causes a speeding of the heart and the other a slowing. A kind of balance between the two systems is constantly in operation. These nerve connections to the brain, however, are not essential for the heartbeat. If all connections to the spine and brain were cut, the heart would still beat, thanks to its own self-contained, independent nerve system.

By counting the pulse or listening with the stethoscope, the physician can usually tell whether the rhythm of the heart is normal or abnormal. For a more precise diagnosis the electrocardiogram is used. This instrument actually records the passage of the electric wave across the chambers of the heart and through the various nerve branches. It is possible to measure the progress of this wave through the heart with great accuracy. The relationship of the electrocardiogram to the activating electric wave is shown in Fig. 2-3. There are a great many abnormalities of the heart rhythm; these will be discussed in a later chapter.

THE FUNCTIONING HEART: THE OXYGEN PUMP

The heart has only one function—to propel blood through the blood vessels. Blood has many functions, but the chief one is to pick up oxygen in the lungs and deliver it to the tisssues of the body. Thus the heart is in effect an oxygen pump.

Use the simple elements of information presented so far and combine them into a picture of the living, functioning heart. Assume some kind of magic vision again that lets you see all the parts of the body. Looking at the heart and great vessels, one sees a torrent of blood rushing from the veins all over the body into the two great cavernous veins and thence into the right atrium, the right top chamber of the heart. The valve between the right atrium and right ventricle swings open, admitting this same gush of blood to the right ventricle, whence it surges through the pulmonary artery into the lungs. The blood that has entered the heart from the veins is dark; this is because it is poor in oxygen, the oxygen having been mostly delivered to the tissues as fuel. In the lungs the blood changes color as it becomes enriched with oxygen, and the blood that flows from the lungs to the left atrium is distinctly bright red in comparison with the rather dark blood emptying from the veins into the right heart. This oxygen-rich blood is then pumped from the left ventricle out to the blood vessels of the entire body.

The heart is contracting rhythmically; first the atria contract, forcing blood down into the ventricles, and then the ventricles contract, the right ventricle emptying its contents into the lungs, the left pumping its load out to the body.

Everything is in a taut balance. The right heart pumps exactly the same volume *into* the lungs that the left pumps *out* with each beat. The valves swing open just in time to admit the rush of blood to the next chamber or out of the heart to the lungs and to the body. They snap shut just in time to prevent a backward rush of blood into the chamber while it is refilling. The observer will notice that the movement of blood through the heart, the lungs, and the vessels of the body is extremely swift. A huge mass of blood (about 6 quarts) moves all around the body from the heart out through the farthest blood vessels, then back through the veins and into the heart again in less than a minute. The synchronized pumping action of the heart muscle, in other words, keeps this torrent of blood moving at a tremendous velocity.

Because the heart and lungs function together as an oxygen intake mechanism, one cannot comprehend the workings of the one without understanding the other; it is important for the reader to learn something of the structure and function of the lungs.

Start with the windpipe, or **trachea,** the ringed tunnel of cartilage that leads from the throat to the chest. This soon divides into two main branches, each called a **bronchus.** The right and left bronchi divide further into smaller and smaller passages, each passage finally ending in a tiny air cell, or **alveolus.** The air passages may be pictured as a bunch of grapes, the stem being the trachea and the grapes representing the alveoli.

In the alveolus you approach a miraculous physical-chemical exchange that is the very buttress of all terrestrial life (Fig. 2-4). Imagine a single alveolus so big that you could stand inside it. In other words, imagine that an alveolus, instead of being microscopic in size, was actually 10 or 15 feet across. You would stand inside a roughly spherical room with a door leading out into a tunnel. Air would come rushing in this tunnel at intervals. The walls of this room would be extremely thin, they would be moist to the touch, and they would be semitransparent. Looking through this wall, you would see a torrent of red fluid pouring past just on the other side. This would be the blood rushing through a capillary that lies immediately across the thin membrane of the alveolus. This capillary would be a branch of the pulmonary artery leading from the right heart. The thin membranous wall of the alveolus and the extremely thin wall of the capillary pressed tightly against it together form a membrane that makes life possible.

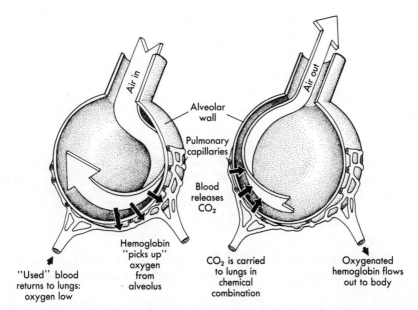

Fig. 2-4. Gas exchange in the lung. Oxygen moves from the lungs into the blood, and carbon dioxide, a waste product, is released from the blood to the lungs, where it is breathed out.

Across this thin, semitransparent, moist membrane, oxygen passes from the air into the blood. Across this membrane in the other direction, carbon dioxide passes from the blood into the alveolus and thence out the tunnel to the trachea. The blood is pouring by in a torrent, like a swiftly rushing river. The exchange of oxygen into the blood and of carbon dioxide out of the blood takes place at an unbelievably rapid rate.

That is well and good. You can picture air being breathed into the air chamber in which we stand and further imagine oxygen moving across the extremely thin, moist membrane that forms the wall of the alveolus. How is oxygen actually carried in the blood? How does a gas like oxygen become part of a liquid like blood?

Oxygen is carried in the blood in two ways: it is either dissolved in the blood or combined with it chemically. Gases do dissolve in liquids, although most of them do not dissolve very well. Everyone who has ever opened a bottle of soda pop has seen a gas coming out of a liquid in which it had been dissolved. When carbon dioxide is put under pressure, it dissolves in the fluid; when the pressure is released by uncapping the bottle, the pressure falls and the carbon dioxide bubbles out. Oxygen does not dissolve as well as carbon dioxide, and if there were no other way for oxygen to enter the blood, life could not continue. The blood contains an amazing substance called hemoglobin, which is carried in the red blood cells. Hemoglobin combines iron with a protein element, globin. This substance can bind, or take on, oxygen and can release it with unbelievable speed. Everyone has seen a rusty tin can. The metal of the tin can has "taken on" oxygen when it formed rust. When iron rusts, for example, it becomes a combination of iron and

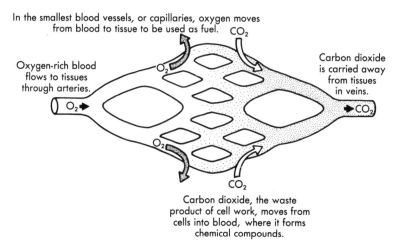

Fig. 2-5. Exchange of oxygen and carbon dioxide in the small blood vessels (capillaries) in the tissues. Oxygen is released into the tissues, and carbon dioxide is carried away.

oxygen, or ferric oxide. Many substances can combine with oxygen in a similar way. Hemoglobin combines with oxygen in a way that is chemically different from the rusting of metal, but the basic concept is the same. Hemoglobin as a substance can combine with oxygen, or take it up, very swiftly. When the hemoglobin has "picked up" oxygen, it becomes oxyhemoglobin. This happens as the blood rushes past the thin membrane of the alveolar wall. The red blood cells are hurled through the left heart and out to the tissues of the body. As the blood percolates through the tissues, the hemoglobin releases its contained oxygen for use as fuel by the cells (Fig. 2-5).

How is the waste product, the carbon dioxide, carried away from the tissues? Carbon dioxide reacts with elements in the blood to form bicarbonate or carbonic acid. Both of these are familiar to you. Soda bicarbonate is what you probably took for an acid stomach or hangover; carbonic acid is the carbon dioxide–containing substance in any carbonated drink, which comes out in bubbles when you open the bottle. These two chemicals "carry" the carbon dioxide just as the hemoglobin carries oxygen. The carbon dioxide enters into one of these two chemical combinations, mostly bicarbonate, out in the tissues; when these chemicals reach the capillaries of the lungs, they release the carbon dioxide into the alveolar chamber. Thus bicarbonate and carbonic acid transport carbon dioxide from tissues to lungs in the same way that hemoglobin carries oxygen from lungs to tissues.

Hemoglobin is almost saturated with oxygen, even when it is exposed to the low concentration of oxygen normally present in the lungs. Breathing 100% oxygen does not increase the amount of oxygen carried by hemoglobin because it is already carrying about as much as it possibly can. When you breathe pure oxygen, you increase the amount of oxygen that is dissolved in the blood in solution, as distinguished from the oxygen carried by the hemoglobin. This increase is small, but it is an increase that may spell the difference between life and death.

The left heart receives the oxygenated blood from the lungs. With each beat some 60 milliliters (about 2 ounces) of blood are pumped to the tissues. Each minute the heart may pump 4 or 5 quarts of blood. During exercise the left ventricle may pump several times this amount, and during sleep the volume will be measurably less. Some organs have huge oxygen requirements; as a result, they need and receive an amount of blood flow much greater than you would imagine, considering their size and weight. Under different conditions of need, the blood vessels to individual organs and tissues contract and expand. This decreases or increases the flow to the individual organs as their need changes.

Back in the alveolus contemplating that moist, pearly membrane and the red torrent rushing by on just the other side of it, it is clear that there are two basic disorders that can block the passage of oxygen from the air to the body. First, there may be some disease of the alveolar wall or of the alveolus itself. That thin, easily permeable membrane may become thick and scarred, posing an impenetrable wall to the passage of air; the alveolus itself may become filled with blood, fluid, or pus so that it cannot function at all; or, finally, whole sections of the lung containing thousands of alveoli may be lost to function because they are destroyed by some disease process such as cancer or inflammation.

There is another possibility. Over on the other side of that transparent membrane in the circulation there may simply not be enough blood rushing past the alveolar surface to pick up adequate amounts of oxygen for the body's needs. This might be the result of inadequate output of blood volume by the heart because the heart is failing, or it could be the result of blockage of one or more of the arteries conducting the blood into the lungs as a result of a blood clot.

Sometimes both sides of the machine fail; in left heart failure the lungs become so engorged with blood that the high pressure in the tiny pulmonary blood vessels forces watery fluid through the alveolar wall, filling the air spaces. The lungs literally become waterlogged because the pressure in the blood vessels is too high and the watery part of the blood "overflows" into the air spaces.

Finally, the blood itself may not be capable of carrying adequate oxygen supplies to the body; anemia may reduce the number of oxygen-carrying red blood cells below a critical level, or poisoning by chemicals like cyanide or carbon monoxide may interfere with the ability of the hemoglobin to pick up oxygen.

Thus a number of diseases of the lungs, the heart, the blood vessels, or the blood itself have one deadly end point in common—failure of delivery of adequate amounts of oxygen to sustain life.

EXERCISE AND THE OXYGEN PUMP

Sitting quietly, the average adult burns about 250 cubic centimeters of oxygen a minute—about a cupful at sea level. With exercise the body's need increases and the oxygen burned per minute may double or triple; trained athletes can increase their oxygen consumption fivefold.

The body can increase its uptake of oxygen by three different mechanisms:
1. More rapid and deeper breathing, increasing the volume of air passing in and out of the lungs.

2. Increased output of blood by the heart (the heart can increase the blood volume pumped per minute in two ways—first, it can beat faster, and second, it can pump more blood with each beat).
3. The body can on demand extract more oxygen from the blood flowing through the lungs.

Everybody knows that with physical training breathing becomes progressively easier at the same level of exercise and the heart does not seem to pound as hard. This is chiefly the result of improvement in **stroke volume,** or the amount of blood pumped with each beat of the heart. In other words, physical training makes the heart a more efficient pump. The trained heart can increase the amount of blood pumped with each beat with increased efficiency and hence does not have to beat as fast to accomplish the same work.

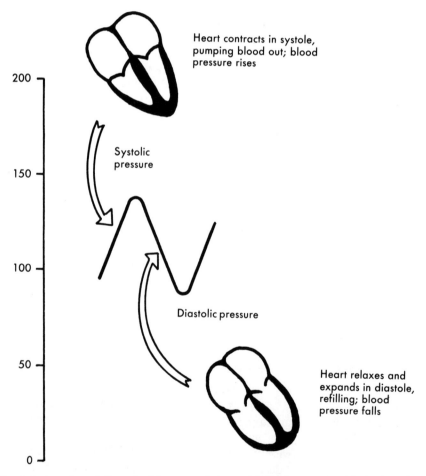

Fig. 2-6. Systole and diastole. The normal rise and fall of pressure with the heartbeat.

As for the other parts of the heart-lung machine, the lungs themselves do not change appreciably with physical training, but some people, particularly gifted athletes, can increase the amount of oxygen extracted from each unit of blood with training. There seems to be an inherited, or genetic, ability to do this in really great athletes who have remarkable endurance. Through some difference in the chemistry of their bodies they can increase the amount of oxygen extracted from each unit of blood as much as fivefold, thereby giving them a remarkable advantage over their fellows.

This section deserves some careful thought and study; understanding the function of the heart as an oxygen pump is essential to any understanding of heart disease, its prevention, and its treatment.

PRESSURES IN THE SYSTEM

A certain pressure is present in the blood vessels of the body at all times. Because the heart is constantly contracting and relaxing, the pressure in the arteries rises and falls with each beat. When the left ventricle is discharging its blood into the arteries, the pressure rises, and between beats while the left ventricle is refilling, the pressure drops (Fig. 2-6). This rise and fall of pressure in the blood vessels with each beat of the heart makes it possible to feel a pulse in the arteries of the wrist or in other vessels of the body. When recording a patient's blood pressure, the physician first measures the top pressure, that is, the pressure when the pulse wave is highest, as illustrated in Fig. 2-6. This is the highest pressure existing within the blood vessels when the left ventricle is ejecting the peak volume of blood into the arteries. The bottom pressure of the pulse curve is also measured. This is the pressure in the arteries when the aortic valve has closed and the left ventricle is refilling. At this point no blood is being pumped out of the heart into the arteries, hence the pressure is relatively low. The pressure is measured in millimeters of mercury. When the physician tells you that your blood pressure is 120 over 80, he means that the top pressure, when the left ventricle is pumping blood into the arteries, is 120 millimeters of mercury and the bottom pressure, between beats when no blood is being pumped, is 80.

The pressure in the pulmonary artery and right ventricle is relatively low— about one fifth the pressure in the left ventricle, the aorta, and the arteries of the body generally. The reader should note this difference and remember it; a rise in pressure in the blood vessels of the lungs is an important feature of many kinds of heart disease.

3   Heart failure

So far this book has pictured the normal functioning heart. You can visualize this living, electrically activated pump as it propels a torrent of blood through the vessels of the body. Everything is in a taut balance; fluid volumes entering and leaving the lungs are exactly the same with each beat of the heart. As you contemplate the heart, you will realize that you are really looking at two pumps, the right heart and the left heart. Each has a different function, and each can be thought of to some extent as a separate unit.

So far these two units, the right heart and left heart, have been described as working together, pumping an identical amount of blood into the lungs and out of them with each beat of the heart. What if this doesn't happen? For example, what if something happens to weaken the left ventricle so that it cannot keep up with the flood of blood rushing into it through the pulmonary veins from the lungs? Any number of diseases might do this. Infections like diphtheria might attack the heart muscle and inflame it, poor blood supply through narrowed or plugged-up coronary arteries might kill some areas of the muscle in the wall of the left ventricle, or diseased valves or high blood pressure might overload the left ventricle past tolerance. For any of these reasons, suppose that the left ventricle pumps a little less blood *out* of the lungs than the right ventricle pumps *in* with each beat. The lungs would soon become congested with blood that would be trapped and could not be expelled through the weakened left ventricle. This is one form of congestive heart failure.

On the other hand, if the right ventricle is weakened in some manner it may not pump the blood from the veins into the lungs as rapidly as the blood is delivered from the veins to the right heart. As a result, congestion will "back up" through the veins of the body, producing watery swelling in the tissues (dropsy). When a physician refers to **congestive heart failure,** he is describing either or both of these conditions, that is, congestion of the lungs with blood because of failure of the left ventricle to drain the blood out of them adequately or back pressure of blood in the veins of the body because of failure of the right ventricle to drain the blood out of the veins efficiently.

Some simple arithmetic will give you a clear idea of what happens in this condition. Suppose the right side of the heart pumps one drop more blood **into the lungs** than the left side of the heart pumps out with each beat. If the heart is beating eighty times a minute, this means that in one or two minutes, 2 teaspoons of blood will be trapped in the lungs. At the same rate in one or two hours a glassful of blood will be trapped in the lungs, above the normal volume that should be present. Within one day the lungs may become so congested with blood that the patient will begin to notice the first symptom of left heart failure—**shortness of breath.** The reason for this is obvious: the lungs are so engorged with blood that there is not enough room for the air to be breathed in and out.

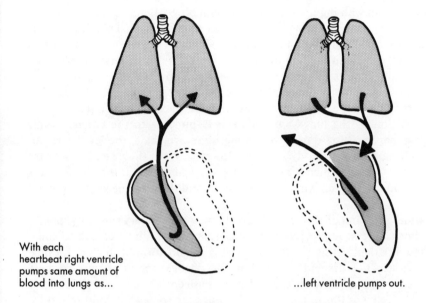

With each heartbeat right ventricle pumps same amount of blood into lungs as...

...left ventricle pumps out.

When left ventricle is diseased, it may pump less blood than normal with each beat.

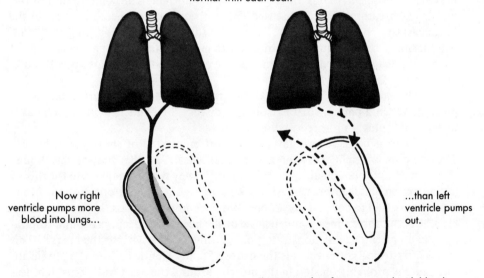

Now right ventricle pumps more blood into lungs...

...than left ventricle pumps out.

Lungs are therefore engorged with blood.

Fig. 3-1. Left heart failure. Congestion of the lungs with blood.

The principal symptom of failure of the left side of the heart is shortness of breath. This kind of shortness of breath may become noticeable during physical exertion. A man walking up a slight hill or climbing a flight of stairs would be forced to stop and pant, much as if he had been running hard. This shortness of breath often appears gradually and progresses slowly. The patient notices that it is more and more difficult for him to carry on various types of physical exertion. The hill or flight of stairs he could climb a year ago now leaves him panting for breath halfway up. After a time he may find that even ordinary light activity, such as walking about the house, produces difficult, panting breathing. The process of congestion of the lungs has been slowly building to the danger point. When the patient is sitting quietly or resting in an armchair, the left heart can pump enough blood for his body's needs. However, when the heart beats faster and pumps more blood, which it must during physical exertion, the diseased left heart simply cannot keep up with the right heart, and the lungs become engorged with blood.

At times this kind of shortness of breath may appear very suddenly. Sometimes it happens late at night. Every physician has made a hurried call to some home to find a patient sitting up in bed, gasping for breath, bluish color on face and lips, obviously in a desperate condition. The deadly process of congestion of the lungs has been going on while the patient was asleep. The heart works under a handicap when one lies flat in bed, since the lungs are somewhat compressed by the upward pressure of the abdominal organs through the diaphragm. Nobody breathes as efficiently lying flat as when sitting upright. The combination of this inefficient breathing with a diseased left ventricle pushes the congestion in the lungs past the "breaking point." The patient suddenly wakens gasping for breath with his lungs barely pumping enough air to maintain life. This particular type of congestive heart failure demands immediate medical attention; it is literally a life-and-death emergency.

The exact kind of shortness of breath produced by left heart failure is important. When a patient suffers from this disease, he pants heavily, exactly as if he had run quickly up three flights of stairs.

Often nervous individuals notice a different kind of shortness of breath. They describe a "tight sensation around their chest," or they may feel as though they "can't take enough air into their lungs." They try to compensate for this by taking extremely deep breaths with a kind of sighing in-and-out motion. Many times I have had to conceal my amusement watching a nervous, hysterical patient breathe about three times as much as he or she needs with deep, profound respirations in an attempt to demonstrate "not getting enough air into the lungs." This is called hysterical dyspnea; it is the cause of many frantic calls to the physician. The cause is probably tension in the muscles around the chest wall. This tightness or tension gives the neurotic patient a sense of compression or of inadequate breathing. He reacts by overbreathing and makes matters much worse. He breathes in more oxygen than he needs and blows off more carbon dioxide than he should. His system is thrown into a state of alkalosis, and various bizarre symptoms follow. The hands may tingle, the muscles of the hands and arms may cramp, and genuine panic often follows. This set of symptoms is called the **hyper-**

ventilation syndrome, since the patient has actually overventilated his blood. You can feel these symptoms yourself by sitting in front of a clock, breathing as deeply and rapidly as possible for three or four minutes; the effect will be surprising. The yardage of unnecessary electrocardiograms recorded on patients suffering from hysterical dyspnea, placed end to end, would doubtless be a statistical marvel.

True left heart failure, however, is characterized by difficult breathing because of the loss of lung capacity. Two of the forms this may take have been described above; others are common. Sometimes the patient in a borderline state will simply notice that he is very wakeful at night; often he feels more comfortable if he props himself on two or three pillows. **Insomnia** of a particular kind may thus be an early symptom of congestive heart failure. (Most insomnia, please note, is caused by nervous tension, excess coffee, guilty consciences, or other less ominous factors, not by heart failure. I would hate to be remembered as the man who started a mass surge of insomniacs to the nearest cardiologist.)

Sudden exertion far beyond the individual's usual level of activity may push a heart with minimal or well-tolerated abnormality beyond its capacity and trip the mechanism of congestive heart failure. The middle-aged, unconditioned hunter scrambling up a ridge in Wyoming, the skier in Colorado, and the jogger who takes up running too abruptly may find themselves victims of a diseased left ventricle that is suddenly pumping against an impossible load, and the deadly mechanism of engorgement of the lungs may go swiftly into action.

Congestion of the lungs with blood is one factor in left heart failure; it is not the only one. The congestion itself seems to trip other abnormal mechanisms in a kind of vicious circle or spiral. Abnormal reflexes begin to work in the nerves that should regulate breathing, and partly as a result of this the breathing becomes rapid, shallow, and inefficient. At this time of all times the patient needs to breathe deeply, slowly, and efficiently; however, these abnormal reflexes will not permit this. It is likely that there is some spasm or constriction of the small airways in the lungs after congestion has reached a certain point. All these factors combine to produce one final effect, which is inadequate delivery of oxygen to the blood and to the tissues. Their sum total may well be catastrophe.

RIGHT HEART FAILURE (Fig. 3-2)

The superior and inferior venae cavae empty a huge volume of blood into the right heart every minute. The right ventricle must pump this blood into the lungs as rapidly as it flows in from these great veins. If it fails to do this, congestion will "back up" into the veins of the body, just as congestion fills the lungs in left heart failure. Any disease of the tissues in the right ventricle can produce failure of the right heart; so can abnormality of the valve leading from the right heart to the lungs. Most commonly right heart failure is produced by some disease in the lungs themselves. Tuberculosis, bronchitis, or other long-standing infections may produce masses of scar tissue that obstruct the flow of blood into the lungs. The right ventricle must then work abnormally hard to force the needed volume of blood through the choked, scarred mass of blood vessels in the lungs. The day

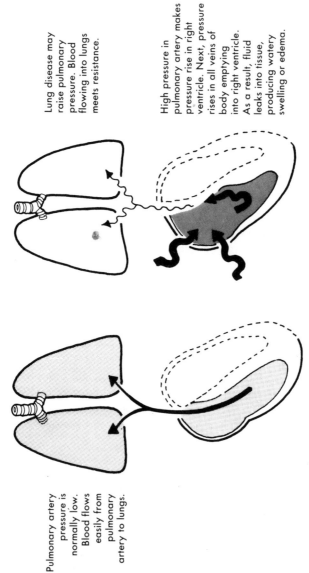

Lung disease may raise pulmonary pressure. Blood flowing into lungs meets resistance.

High pressure in pulmonary artery makes pressure rise in right ventricle. Next, pressure rises in all veins of body emptying into right ventricle. As a result, fluid leaks into tissue, producing watery swelling or edema.

Pulmonary artery pressure is normally low. Blood flows easily from pulmonary artery to lungs.

Fig. 3-2. Right heart failure. High pressure in the pulmonary artery and its branches and in the right heart. This is commonly a result of lung disease.

comes when the right ventricle fails. In this case the congestion fills the veins of the body rather than the blood vessels in the lungs. As the result of greatly increased pressure in the veins, clear watery fluid oozes into the tissues. This fluid is actually a kind of filtered blood; it is a form of water with dissolved salt and other chemical elements, not very different from seawater. The presence of this kind of watery fluid in the tissues is called **edema;** the common term for it is **dropsy.**

Water flows downhill anywhere, even inside the human body. If there is much edema fluid in the tissues, it tends to run down toward the feet or the ankles, particularly if the patient has been standing or walking. This swelling may be quite impressive; sometimes the ankles seem as big around as a small tree trunk when there is a good deal of edema fluid present. Without treatment the swelling tends to move upward so that the legs and thighs in turn become distended with fluid. Edema fluid may also ooze into the abdominal cavity, and sometimes the abdomen becomes hugely distended. The medical term for this phenomenon is **ascites.** Abnormal back pressure in the veins of the liver will cause that organ to become distended and enlarged.

Right heart failure, to sum up, *is a state of watery swelling, or edema, in the tissues of the body caused by failure of the right ventricle in its task of pumping the blood out of the veins and into the lungs.* Specific causes of right heart failure and methods of treating it will be discussed in later chapters. Often both left and right heart failure may be present at the same time.

If you have a good grasp of these two basically simple phenomena you will have little difficulty understanding the material presented in the rest of this book.

4 The electrocardiogram and what it tells

The electrocardiogram is one of the four or five basic elements of all cardiac diagnoses. Electrocardiographic interpretations are so fundamental to many of the critical decisions of cardiac care that the patient must know something about the technique to participate intelligently in those decisions.

In Chapter 2 the electric activation of the heart is described. The reader without other special medical background should probably review that material at this point.

Briefly, the heart beats because a wave of electric energy is generated in a small cluster of nerve-like cells near the top of the right atrium. These cells perform exactly the same role as the coil in the engine of your car—they actually generate an electric potential and send it out across the conducting tissues of the heart.

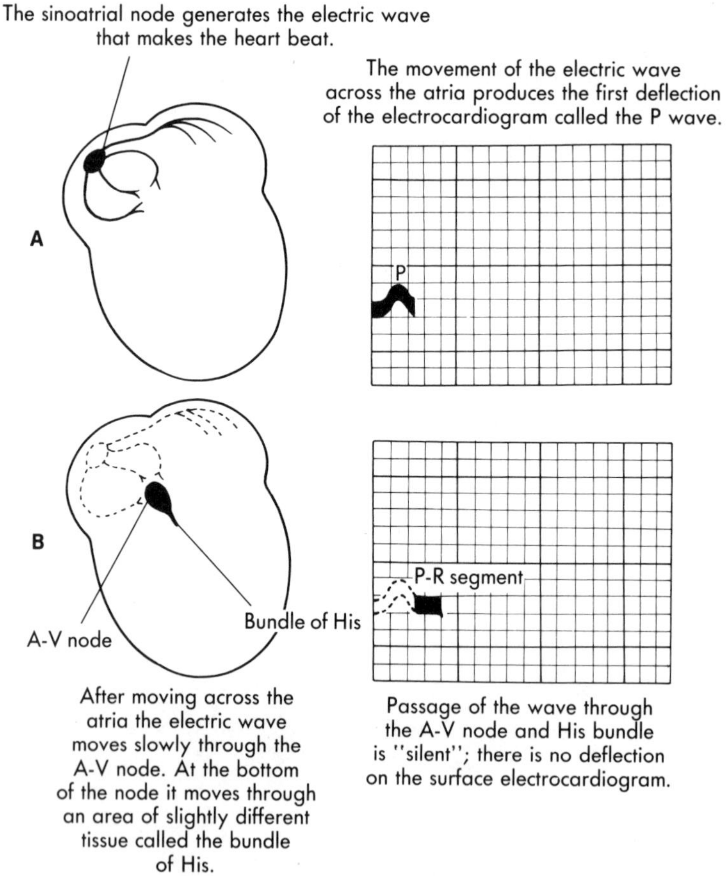

The sinoatrial node generates the electric wave that makes the heart beat.

The movement of the electric wave across the atria produces the first deflection of the electrocardiogram called the P wave.

A

P

B

A-V node

Bundle of His

After moving across the atria the electric wave moves slowly through the A-V node. At the bottom of the node it moves through an area of slightly different tissue called the bundle of His.

P-R segment

Passage of the wave through the A-V node and His bundle is "silent"; there is no deflection on the surface electrocardiogram.

Fig. 4-1. A and **B,** Relationship of the waves of the electrocardiogram to the electric activation of the heart.

It is relatively simple to record the passage of this wave of electric energy. Several electrodes are attached to the body's surface and connected to a recording galvanometer, which moves a pointer up and down, depending on the positive or negative charges being recorded. When the patient is lying quietly, there is no other electric activity in the body in the same frequency range, and hence the electric signal coming from the heart will be easy to detect.

Physicians have agreed on certain standard positions of electrodes on the body surface that seem to give the best picture of the passage of the activating waves through the chambers of the heart. Fig. 4-1 illustrates the course of the activating wave of electric energy through the structures of the heart. The conducting system of the heart is really quite simple; it only has the following four elements:

1. Sinoatrial node—the collection of cells near the top of the right atrium that acts as the generator, or coil, for the heart.
2. The conducting tissues of the atria—a number of fibers lead the activating wave out through both top chambers, much like a ripple spreading across a pond.
3. The atrioventricular (AV) node–His bundle complex—this is a structure

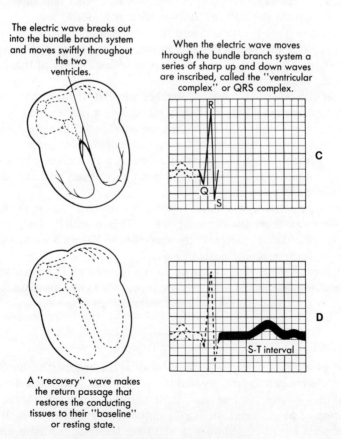

The electric wave breaks out into the bundle branch system and moves swiftly throughout the two ventricles.

When the electric wave moves through the bundle branch system a series of sharp up and down waves are inscribed, called the "ventricular complex" or QRS complex.

C

A "recovery" wave makes the return passage that restores the conducting tissues to their "baseline" or resting state.

S-T interval

D

Fig. 4-1, cont'd. C and **D,** Electric activation of the ventricles.

rather like an outlet canal, or connecting nerve; it conducts the wave of electric energy from atria to ventricles and hence is logically called the atrioventricular node. At the bottom of the node is a small bundle of specialized conducting tissues that extends down into the ventricles; it is named for its discoverer, a German physiologist named His.

4. From the bottom of the bundle of His, two large nerve-like structures course on through the ventricles, one to the right ventricle, one to the left. Because these are branches of the bundle of His, they are called "bundle branches." The left bundle branch carries the activating impulse to the left ventricle, and the right to the right ventricle. The fibers branch out rather like twigs on a tree, ending in tiny nerve fibrils called Purkinje fibers.

Movement of the activating wave from the sinoatrial node across the atria produces the first deflection on the electrocardiogram, which is called the P wave. (The letter "P" wasn't chosen for any particular reason; it could just as well have been X, Y, or Z.)

Passage of the wave down the connecting atrioventricular node between atria and ventricles does not produce any deflection in the surface electrocardiogram; there is a flat segment without electric activity that tells how long it takes the impulse to move through the atrioventricular node.

The wave front breaks out into the two bundle branches and moves very swiftly to activate the ventricles; this movement produces a tall, complicated, spiked wave, the "ventricular complex." The various waves of this complex are named Q, R, and S.

After the outgoing wave has reached the end of the ventricles there is a momentary lull, or quiet period. This is marked by a flat segment in the electrocardiogram because, again, just as during the passage through the AV node, there is no electrical activity to record in the surface electrocardiogram. This short interval is very important in the study of coronary artery disease because it is the one time in the heart cycle when injured heart muscle can be detected by a small current called an "injury current."

Finally, a recovery wave, or T wave, moves back across the heart in the opposite direction from the outgoing wave. This is usually low, upright, and rounded; variations and changes in the shape of the T wave are often very important clues to the presence of heart disease.

What can the physician tell with such a recording? The electrocardiogram gives an amazing amount of information; it probably gives more useful information than any other instrument used in cardiac diagnosis.

HEART RHYTHMS

The physician can diagnose the rhythm of the heart with complete accuracy with the electrocardiogram. By looking at the atrial waves and the ventricular waves and their relation to one another, the physician can tell whether a normal beat is arising in the atria and moving down the usual pathway through the ventricles. If the atria have stopped beating and have begun to fibrillate, there will be no P wave; instead, there will be a fine series of rapid twitching movements in the electrocardiogram. If the atria are fluttering, large sawtooth waves will appear. If there is a block in the atrioventricular node, the physician can detect this by noticing how long it takes the wave to move through this node and can also tell if the wave is blocked so that it does not come through at all. If a paroxysmal tachycardia begins, the physician can tell which chamber the tachycardia originates in, a matter of great clinical importance.

In brief, a skilled electrocardiographer should be able to diagnose abnormalities of the heart rhythm with about 100% accuracy.

CHAMBER ENLARGEMENT

If the activating wave is moving over a huge heart chamber, it will produce a different pattern than a wave moving over a normal heart chamber. For this reason the physician is able to detect enlargement of any of the chambers of the heart by changes in the electrocardiogram. If the enlargement is in the atria, the P waves, or atrial waves, will be abnormal. If the enlargement is in the ventricles, various changes will take place in the ventricular waves. By reasoning out the pattern of enlargement, the physician can deduce many other facts about the heart. Certain kinds of enlargement, taken together with certain abnormal heart sounds, mean that a particular kind of congenital abnormality of the heart is present. Certain kinds of chamber enlargement will also be found in certain kinds of valve disease. Detection of enlargement of one or more chambers of the heart is one of the most important bits of information yielded by the electrocardiogram.

CORONARY DISEASE

If tissue in the heart wall is injured or dead, changes will almost always take place in the electrocardiogram. The dead or injured tissue gives rise to an electric pattern that is different from healthy tissue. These changes will be seen either in the shape of the ventricular wave, by changes in the normally flat S-T segment following the ventricular wave, or by changes in the shape of the recovery, or T, wave. Analysis of these changes is a matter for experts. You must remember two facts, however. First, the electrocardiographer cannot always tell at once what has happened in the heart muscle. If a coronary artery has plugged up, causing death of heart muscle, it may take three or four days for the diagnostic pattern to emerge in the electrocardiogram. Second, sometimes the changes in the electrocardiogram must be called **nonspecific;** this means that there is some abnormality of the recovery, or T, wave that might be caused by any of a dozen different diseases of the heart muscle. The electrocardiogram here tells only that some abnormality is present. The physician must arrive at the cause by other diagnostic means.

On the positive side, the electrocardiogram often permits diagnosis of stoppage of a coronary artery within minutes of the occurrence. The diagnostic accuracy of this instrument is frequently fantastic. It also permits the physician to localize the area of stoppage with some accuracy. (In Chapter 6 the specific alteration seen with the various manifestations of coronary artery disease are described in much greater detail.)

SERUM MINERAL CHANGES

Changes in the mineral elements of the blood such as sodium, potassium, and calcium produce fairly characteristic changes in the electrocardiogram. Sometimes the electrocardiogram is more accurate than an actual blood test in finding abnormality of these elements because they all play a role in the normal function of the heart tissues.

INFLAMMATIONS OF THE HEART

There are many kinds of inflammation of the heart in its various layers (Chapter 13). Any of the inflammations of the heart muscle, whether caused by rheumatic fever, viral infections, bacterial infections, or degenerations of unknown cause, will usually produce some change in the electrocardiogram. These changes are not diagnostic, and the physician cannot look at the electrocardiogram and say, "This patient has pneumococcal infection of the heart muscle." Taking the change in the electrocardiogram, together with other laboratory and clinical findings, however, the physician can state that progressive acute change is going on in the heart muscle and by swift process of deduction and elimination can usually arrive at an accurate diagnosis. Just as in coronary disease it is often necessary to record electrocardiograms every day or two for a period of time to follow the changes in the electric pattern. One tracing often does not tell the story; *diagnosis is based on change in pattern rather than on a particular appearance.*

PERICARDITIS

Inflammation of the sac of tissue around the heart, or pericarditis, usually produces change in the electrocardiogram. In most cases this change is so characteristic that the physician can diagnose the disease and distinguish it from the changes caused by blocking of a coronary artery with death of heart muscle. Again, it will often be necessary to study the changes over a period of two, three, or more days to make this differentiation.

STRESS TESTING

"I once knew a man who had an electrocardiogram, and the doctor told him it was normal. He walked out of the door of the building, and by that night, he was dead of a heart attack. How about that?" Everyone has heard this story. It is perfectly possible. The electrocardiogram is not a crystal ball. It cannot predict what is going to happen to the heart. It can only record what has already happened. Unless actual injury or death of heart muscle has already occurred, the electrocardiogram may be normal, even though there is partial blockage of coronary arteries. It isn't until the blockage goes so far that changes take place in the cells of the heart muscle that the electrocardiogram will begin to alter its appearance.

In the past few years, stress testing has actually increased the accuracy of the electrocardiogram in coronary disease; it now almost does some predicting. The electrocardiogram can be recorded during and after strenuous exercise, when the heart is driven to work at its peak capacity. If blood flow through the coro-

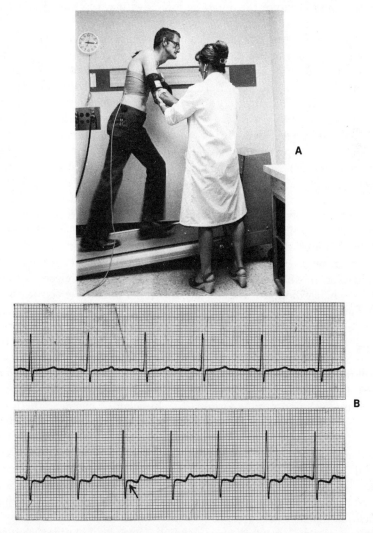

Fig. 4-2. A, Typical treadmill with subject connected to three-channel recorder. Progressive exercise includes increases in speed and elevation of the treadmill. **B,** Electrocardiographic changes during stress testing. Top strip is a normal tracing recorded before exercise. Bottom strip was recorded during anginal pain that had been produced by walking on a treadmill. The depressed, downsloping S-T segment indicates that an area of heart muscle is not receiving an adequate blood supply; this implies disease of the coronary arteries.

nary arteries is partly cut down, it is quite likely that the electrocardiogram will record changes from the areas of heart muscle that are not receiving an adequate blood flow for their increase in work.

When heart muscle does not receive enough blood for its needs, it generates an abnormal, small electric potential called an "injury current." The point in the electric heart cycle when this tiny current can be recorded is during the quiet period between the end of the outgoing, or activating, wave and the beginning of the returning, or restoring, wave of the heart cycle. This interval is called the S-T interval, and observation of it is critical to stress testing. Vital decisions about the presence of coronary artery disease or the need for coronary artery surgery are based on observation of this segment during exercise (Fig. 4-2). Exercise testing, as it is called, is an exceedingly useful procedure; it is a major advance that permits the physician to diagnose coronary artery disease in its early, rather than its late stages (Fig. 4-2).

The standard test first used in exercise testing was the Master test in which the patient walked up and down a small set of stairs of a standard height a given number of times, depending on the patient's age, height, and weight. The patient was then quickly placed on the examining table, and the electrocardiogram was recorded at intervals. This was a very useful test and, in fact, was the first real step forward in studying with the electrocardiogram the effects of physical stress on the heart. Techniques of stress testing have advanced. Now the cardiologist can actually watch the electrocardiogram while the patient carries on various levels of exercise. Light electrodes are pasted on various parts of the body and attached to long, flexible cables plugged into multiple-channel electrocardiographic machines. The cardiologist can actually watch a number of electrocardiographic leads while the patient exercises vigorously on a treadmill or pedals a bicycle against electrical resistance. With a continuous record of the electrocardiogram, the pulse rate, and the blood pressure during exercise of various degrees the cardiologist is in a better position that ever before to detect abnormalities of the coronary arteries and to estimate the total efficiency of the patient's heart in terms of the work the patient can perform.

Stress testing not only permits the physician to diagnose the presence of partial obstruction of the coronary arteries, it can also give some idea of the severity of the coronary artery disease and may be the critical factor in deciding whether medical or surgical treatment is warranted. If a patient walking on a treadmill feels cardiac pain or manifests an injury current at a very low level of exertion, the implication is that the disease is much more severe than if symptoms appeared or an injury current became manifest only at the most strenuous effort of which the patient is capable.

Stress testing is not infallible; sometimes patients with significant coronary disease will produce a normal stress test, while, on the other hand, people with normal coronary arteries may show abnormalities during stress testing. These specifics will be explored further in Chapter 6, Coronary Artery Disease.

5 The cardiac arrhythmias

The rhythm and rate of the heart respond to the needs of the body like a furnace responding to a set of thermostats. With exercise the normal heart speeds, while during a period of reduced need such as sleep the heart rate can become very slow—often less than 50 beats a minute.

The heartbeat is not always regular, even in a healthy person. Count the pulse in your own wrist and note its steady rhythm. Take a deep breath and then exhale. Often the rate will speed during inspiration and slow at the end of expiration. This change in rhythm with breathing is called **sinus arrhythmia;** the name means that this is still a normal rhythm generated by the sinoatrial node, the normal pacemaker of the heart. The changes in rate with breathing are a reflection of the changes in the blood gases percolating through the base of the brain. It is a normal finding.

The heart has a remarkable "fail-safe" system in its conducting tissues. If the sinoatrial node failed to discharge or did not discharge often enough for the body's needs or if the exciting impulse was blocked by diseased tissue in its passage from atria to ventricles, the heart could still beat because of the hundreds of "reserve pacemakers," or ectopic foci, scattered through all chambers of the heart—through the atria, the atrioventricular (AV) node, and the ventricles. Any one of these minute areas of tissue is capable of generating a heartbeat and properly does so when the normal pacemaker fails to fire or is blocked. In other words, these "reserve pacemakers" are in the heart for a very good reason.

Sometimes, however, one of the reserve pacemakers becomes "irritable"; this can happen as a result of chemical irritation from nicotine or caffeine, emotional tension, or any of a number of disease states. Almost everybody has felt a sensation at one time or another as though the heart "skipped a beat" or "turned over and hung still for a second." What has happened is that one of these pacemakers has fired a beat, interrupting the normal sinus rhythm of the heart, even though it wasn't needed. These beats are called **ectopic** beats, since they arise outside the normal site. (The word "ectopic" in medicine refers to something that takes place where it shouldn't; thus an ectopic pregnancy is a pregnancy in a tube instead of in the uterus, etc.) The extra, or ectopic, beat (Fig. 5-1) comes soon after the normal beat, like this:

BEAT   BEAT   BEATbeat   BEAT

There is usually a pause in the rhythm after the extra beat. The next normal beat comes when it would have if there had been no break in the rhythm, that is, if there had been a normal beat where it should have been, right in the middle of the pause. This temporary pause in the heartbeat often gives a feeling as if the heart had stopped beating. It can be frightening, but it has no real meaning; the heart always starts again.

Sometimes these extra beats come often, even every other beat, like this:

BEATbeat   BEATbeat   BEATbeat   BEATbeat

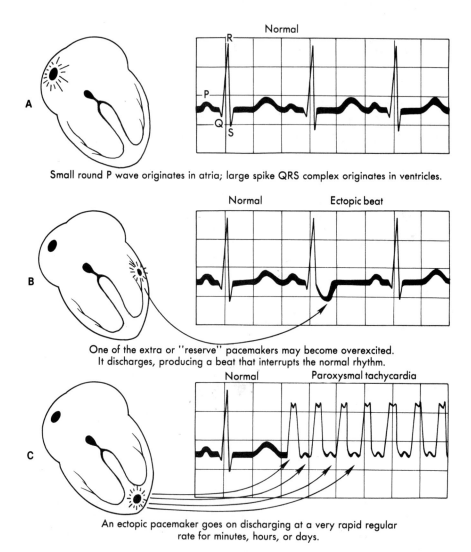

Small round P wave originates in atria; large spike QRS complex originates in ventricles.

One of the extra or "reserve" pacemakers may become overexcited.
It discharges, producing a beat that interrupts the normal rhythm.

An ectopic pacemaker goes on discharging at a very rapid regular
rate for minutes, hours, or days.

Fig. 5-1. A, Sinus, or normal rhythm. **B,** Single ectopic beat. **C,** Sustained or continuous firing—ectopic tachycardia.

When premature beats come in a regular rhythm, the physician will want to check for increased irritability of heart tissues; this might be caused by medication, disease, or a variety of reasons. Remember, however, occasional premature beats have no real significance, they do not imply heart disease. If they occur often or in a regular pattern, the physician will probably want to investigate further.

PAROXYSMAL TACHYCARDIA

The name of this arrhythmia is impressive; actually, it is very simple. Without any warning the heart suddenly begins to race, beating 200 or 300 times a minute. This is a perfectly regular rhythm. The heart pounds like a swiftly pumping machine, while the patient wonders what the terrifying sensation is in his chest. (The word "paroxysm" in medical usage means anything that starts and stops suddenly; "tachycardia" means any heart rate over 100 beats per minute.)

What has happened? If you understand the section on premature beats, you will understand paroxysmal tachycardia. One of the same extra, or ectopic, pacemakers that causes ectopic beats has begun firing these beats continuously (Fig. 5-1, C). The pacemaker **goes on firing** for minutes, hours, or days, driving the heart at a very rapid rate. The attack can come on while the patient is sitting quietly, eating, driving a car, for no apparent reason. It starts like this:

BEAT   BEAT   BEATbeatbeatbeatbeatbeatbeatbeatbeat

and so on for an indefinite period.

The patient always knows when a paroxysmal tachycardia starts. The very rapid, pounding heartbeat is frightening. Often the patient will find it hard to breathe or will feel a sense of oppression in the chest.

As a rule, a heart can beat rapidly like this for hours or even one or two days with no great harm. However, if this rapid action goes on for several days, the heart may begin to fail. Beating so rapidly, the heart does not have time to fill properly between beats. (Imagine trying to fill a bulb syringe with water and squeezing it out 300 or 400 times per minute. There wouldn't be time for the syringe to fill properly before it was squeezed the next time.) The amount of blood pumped per minute falls, and congestive heart failure may result.

Sometimes these tachycardias stop for no reason, just as they start. More often, medical care is needed. Various drugs can be used. It is curious, however, that the kind of treatment will depend on the location of the abnormal pacemaker in the heart. If the paroxysmal tachycardia is caused by a pacemaker in the atria or in a connecting node between atria and ventricles, one group of cardiac medications may be used effectively and safely. If the tachycardia is caused by a pacemaker in the ventricles, an entirely different group of drugs will be used. What is good treatment for tachycardia coming from the "top" of the heart may be ineffective or dangerous for tachycardia arising in the "bottom." The physician must make a precise diagnosis of the kind of paroxysmal tachycardia. This can be done only with an electrocardiogram.

What is the significance of paroxysmal tachycardia? Does it mean the heart is diseased? Every patient wants to know the answers to these questions as soon as the racing has been stopped. Again, a curious difference exists.

If the tachycardia arises in the atria or in the atrioventricular node, it does not necessarily imply organic heart disease. This kind of tachycardia is often found in people with perfectly normal hearts. They may have attacks of tachycardia all their lives and die at the age of 92 with normal hearts. Patients do occasionally have attacks every few weeks all their lives, but usually no cause is found, and they live out a normal life span.

If the tachycardia arises in the ventricles—in the "bottom" of the heart—there is almost sure to be some kind of heart disease present. This might be mild or severe, acute or chronic, but some organic abnormality of the heart is practically always the cause. The physician will want to make a careful search for it. The physician can usually control or prevent these attacks since a whole battery of drugs and methods are available to choose from, but—a warning—the patient must be patient! A great deal of careful testing and adjusting must go on; no two patients ever respond to the same dose of the same drug in the same way.

In extreme cases that resist drug treatment electric countershock can be used safely and effectively. In this dramatic advance in heart treatment an instantaneous shock is delivered by means of an automatic control during the "safe" period of the heart cycle; a normal heartbeat is almost always the result. This calls for expensive equipment and experienced physicians, but the equipment and the personnel to do this are now available in almost every major hospital in the country. Electric shock to stop paroxysmal tachycardia has been a tremendous advance in treatment, and the procedure saves lives every day.

ATRIAL FIBRILLATION

Again imagine that you can see a beating heart. The atria contract and then the ventricles in a regular rhythm, top-bottom, top-bottom, atria-ventricles, atria-ventricles.

Suddenly the atria stop their regular beat. They begin a fine, fast, twitching movement. The surface of the atrial chambers is crisscrossed by many tiny waves of contraction moving in all directions, looking much like the surface of a still pond after handfuls of pebbles are flung into it. This irregular, rapid twitching is called "fibrillation" (Fig. 5-2).

The ventricles, remember, continue to contract, pumping the blood to the lungs and to the body. Only the atria suddenly go into this twitching kind of abnormal movement. However, the observer will notice quickly that the beat of the ventricles soon becomes irregular. The great chambers continue to pump blood, but they lose the steady beat, beat, beat, of a normal heart rhythm. Some of the ventricular beats will come close together, some far apart, and there will be runs of rapic beats and periods of slow ones. The rhythm suddenly doesn't make any sense.

Remember that in normal conduction an electric wave moves down the atrioventricular node and into the ventricles each time the atria contract. When the atria fibrillate, there is no such regular movement. Instead, the hundreds of fine electric impulses crisscrossing the atria bombard the atrioventricular node like sparks from a pinwheel. Those that happen to arrive when the atrioventricular node is ready to conduct will reach the ventricles and produce a beat. Many will arrive at the node when it cannot conduct because it has just passed a beat through, and these following beats will be blocked. The ventricular beat will become completely helter-skelter with no regular rhythm. The pulse will feel something like this:

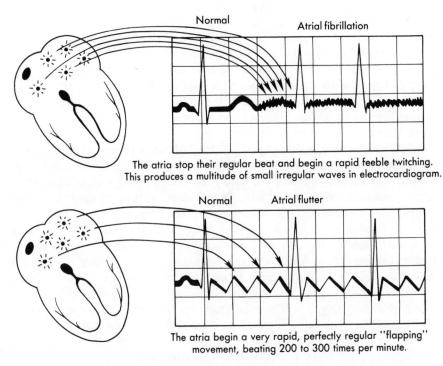

Normal   Atrial fibrillation

The atria stop their regular beat and begin a rapid feeble twitching.
This produces a multitude of small irregular waves in electrocardiogram.

Normal   Atrial flutter

The atria begin a very rapid, perfectly regular "flapping"
movement, beating 200 to 300 times per minute.

Fig. 5-2. Atrial fibrillation and atrial flutter.

BEAT   beat   beatbeat   BEAT   beat   BEAT
                    beat   beat   BEAT   BEAT

Delirium cordis, delirium of the heart, was the name physicians once gave
to this irregularity. Before medical therapy was available, the irregular heartbeat
often drove the heart into fatal congestive failure.

Why does this happen? There are a number of reasons. A diseased heart
valve that causes the atria to enlarge and blow up something like a small balloon
is a common cause. For this reason, **mitral stenosis** is probably the most common
cause of atrial fibrillation, since the left atrium becomes hugely enlarged above
the narrow valve opening. Disease of the coronary arteries, which supply the
atrial muscle, can also cause fibrillation. The scarred, dead tissue produced by
lack of blood flow is the trigger in these cases. Whatever the cause, the presence
of electrically "dead" tissue in the atria seems to set up a "short circuit" that
detonates the electric explosion. The normal progressive activating wave is shat-
tered into a mass of self-perpetuating electric circuits, and the tissues are driven to
fibrillate. An overactive thyroid gland can also start the atria fibrillating. The excess of thyroid hormone seems to make the heart tissues unusually irritable, and
fibrillation follows.

Atrial fibrillation is dangerous for two reasons. First, the heartbeat becomes inefficient and congestive failure may follow. The hit-or-miss stimulation of the ventricles finds these chambers filled only partially at the time they are driven to contract. They may be half full or a third full in comparison with the amount of blood ready for ejection with a normal, coordinated heartbeat. The beat becomes inefficient, meaning less blood is pumped per minute. Any time the volume of blood pumped per minute falls very much, the deadly chain reaction of congestive heart failure may be set in motion.

Second, the atria do not expel their load of blood completely and cleanly. There is **stagnation** in the recesses of these chambers. When blood stagnates, it clots. The clots, rather like lumps of hard jelly, attach to the walls of the atria. If the atrial fibrillation goes on for months and years, as it often does, these clots may break off in lumps and bits, and they are then pumped out into the circulation. A clot floating through the arteries is like a fused time bomb. Within a matter of seconds it will float into an artery that is too small to let it pass; the clot then plugs the artery completely, and the tissue that depends on that artery for its blood supply will die. If this happens in the brain, paralysis or death may follow. If an artery is stopped up in either leg, gangrene and amputation lie ahead. Wherever the clot stops, it will plug an artery and cut off blood supply to some area of the body. With luck, this will be a small artery to an area that doesn't matter very much. Very often, however, the patient is not this lucky. A large artery to some vital organ is stopped up, and the result is a disaster of some degree. This kind of discharge of a clot into the arteries of the body happens in about one third of all cases of chronic artrial fibrillation.

Atrial fibrillation can be attacked in several ways. First, the wild, erratic, rapid ventricular beat can be slowed and the patient brought quickly out of congestive failure. Digitalis does this; in carefully regulated doses the drug slows conduction through the atrioventricular node. It cuts down the number of impulses reaching the ventricles each minute. The ventricular rhythm is still irregular, but the beat is now slower and more efficient. The heart can pump the lungs clear of congestion, and the patient will be able to breathe normally. This effect is dramatic. A patient who enters a hospital gasping for air and near death may be strolling about the corridors comfortably within twenty-four hours.

Second, the fibrillation itself can be stopped and a normal beat restored to the atria. The physician can do this by administering a drug, quinidine, under close, careful supervision. Like all useful medical agents, quinidine is powerful; an overdose may be harmful. The physician will check pulse, blood pressure, and electrocardiographic change while attempting to restore a normal rhythm in the atria. This is not something to do casually at home or while going about one's daily round of work or play.

If quinidine fails to restore a normal atrial rhythm, electric shocks may succeed. This is the same kind of electric shock described in the section of paroxysmal tachycardia; it must be delivered by an electronic system linked to the patient's own electrocardiogram. The timing of this shock is a life-and-death matter; it must come during the "safe" period of the heart cycle. The shock must be very brief—about fifteen thousandths of a second—and it must be of a certain controlled intensity. All these variable factors are controlled by a machine developed by Dr. Lown and his associates at Harvard University Medical School. Electric restoration of normal heartbeat has become a matter of pressing a button. A shock of the right duration, intensity, and timing flashes through the heart, triggered by the patient's own electrocardiogram. The regular beep-beep-beep of a normal heartbeat on the sound element of a cardiac monitor is becoming the most beautiful sound in the world to those cardiologists who work with this remarkable machine.

The best treatment of this arrhythmia is removal of the cause. If a diseased valve can be corrected by surgery or if an overactive thyroid can be suppressed medically or removed by the surgeon, the arrhythmia often disappears forever.

If atrial fibrillation persists despite all these measures, the physician will usually consider giving anticoagulants—drugs that prevent clots from forming. Frequent blood checks are needed when these drugs are used, but the danger more than justifies the trouble. Better a blood test every month than a blood clot in the brain!

ATRIAL FLUTTER

Atrial flutter is an arrhythmia that is a kind of "second cousin" to atrial fibrillation. Instead of twitching irregularly, the atria go into a very rapid flapping movement (Fig. 5-2, *B*) like the wings of a bird, beating with perfect regularity 200 to 300 times a minute. Usually the connecting node between atria and ventricles cannot conduct this fast. Only every other atrial beat or every third or fourth beat can travel through to the ventricles. The physician will describe a flutter as "two to one," "four to one," or "six to one," depending on the number of atrial beats for each ventricular beat. One could picture a two to one flutter like this:

Atria	BEAT		BEAT		BEAT		BEAT		BEAT		BEAT	
Ventricles		BEAT				BEAT					BEAT	

The causes of atrial flutter are largely the same as the causes of atrial fibrillation. Treatment is different, however. The physician will always want to verify this diagnosis with an electrocardiogram.

Sometimes these rapid irregularities of the heartbeat make a patient feel as though his chest were congested as in a common cold. I have had a patient ask for a prescription for a "chest cold" over the telephone; on examination, the man actually suffered from rapid atrial flutter, which no amount of aspirin or nose drops could have helped.

ATRIOVENTRICULAR BLOCK

The atrioventricular node is the only normal connection between the atria and the ventricles. The cells in this node must be healthy, functioning units or transmission down the vital channel falters. Many diseases attack these cells. Acute rheumatic heart disease, diphtheritic heart disease, viral infections of the heart, and degeneration of the tissues because of poor coronary blood supply may all affect transmission through the atrioventricular node. When the cells of the atrioventricular node are significantly diseased, some form of block in this node will appear. This is usually what a physician means by **heart block.**

In the mildest form of atrioventricular block the activating wave takes longer than it should to travel from atria down to ventricles (Fig. 5-3, *A*). The difference from normal transmission time may be only a few hundredths of a second. This kind of block can be detected only by an electrocardiogram.

At other times the cells in the atrioventricular node conduct so slowly that only every other atrial beat or every third or fourth atrial beat can pass through. Now the patient may suffer some symptoms. The beat of the ventricles may be very slow, and sudden attacks of faintness or dizziness may appear.

Finally, the cells in the atrioventricular node may lose all function; they are, in effect, dead. They are often replaced by inert scar tissue that cannot transmit an activating wave. No beats at all can travel from atria to ventricles. Life is maintained by one of the "extra" pacemakers in the ventricles that goes into action and begins setting the beat. This is **complete** heart block (Fig. 5-3, *B*). The atria and the ventricles now beat independently of each other, and there is no longer any functional connection between the top and bottom of the heart as far as rhythm goes.

When heart block of severe degree slows the ventricles, a frightening kind of seizure may follow. The ventricles may actually stop for a few seconds, blood flow to the brain may fall below the amount needed to maintain consciousness, and the patient falls in a faint or convulsion. Such episodes are usually brief; as a rule, the ventricles take up a beat and consciousness is restored without any medical treatment. These seizures are called Stokes-Adams attacks, named for the two great Irish physicians of the eighteenth century who first described them.

Until recently treatment with various drugs was the only way to control these dangerous attacks. Drug treatment was helpful in some cases but of little value in others. Electric pacing of the heart, however, has now become quite simple and very practical. By means of electric stimulators the heart can be run at a normal rate for years, probably as long as desired. If a slow rate is endangering the patient's life, the heart can be driven in an emergency by inserting a long, thin, flexible, wire electrode into it, either through the chest wall by means of a needle or up a vein from either arm, threading the wire around through the top of the chest, and down into the right ventricle. This wire is then attached to an electric pacer, and by twisting a couple of knobs the intensity and rate of the heartbeat are electrically controlled. This sounds formidable and complicated, but actually it is such a simple procedure that it can be carried out in almost any hospital in the United States. With the heart beating at a reasonable rate, the patient's life is no longer in danger. If the block persists, surgery can then be performed so that a very tiny electric pacer, consisting of an unbelievably small battery and timing device, can actually be implanted inside the chest wall with wires attached to the heart. Again, this has a kind of science fiction ring to it, but the procedure is not technically difficult, and the electric pacers that have been developed in the last few years are fantastically efficient. The operation of implanting such a pace-

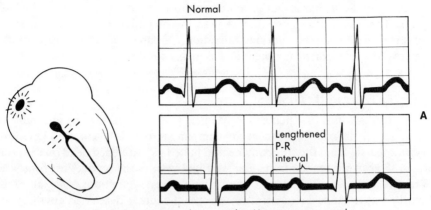

Each wave from atria reaches ventricles. However, a wave takes a long time passing through diseased atrioventricular node.

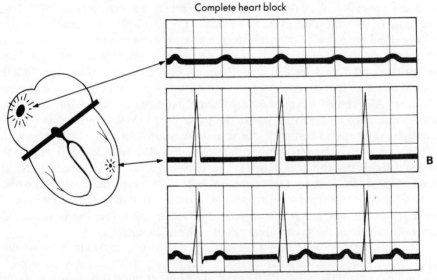

Cells in atrioventricular node are dead and impulses cannot pass from atria to ventricles. Atria and ventricles beat independently, ventricles being driven by an ectopic pacemaker (same kind of pacemaker that produces premature beats).

Fig. 5-3. A, Each wave from atria reaches ventricles. However, a wave takes a long time passing through diseased atrioventricular node. **B,** Cells in atrioventricular node are dead and impulses cannot pass from atria to ventricles. Atria and ventricles beat independently, ventricles being driven by an ectopic pacemaker (same kind of pacemaker that produces premature beats).

maker is not difficult and can be done in almost any major hospital in the United States. The results are spectacular. A man wearing an artificial pacemaker in his heart is in most respects a normal individual. He can go about the business of living free of the terror of a violent and possibly fatal seizure.

FATAL ARRHYTHMIAS

In 1942, as a first lieutenant, Medical Corps, I was jogging at double time to the motor park at the head of my company in the 12th Armored Division. A cry and scuffle from the company behind halted us. Stretched dead on the ground was a 35-year-old former bartender who had been in the service just four weeks. Why did the man die? In accordance with army regulations, a "line of duty board" was organized to determine whether the man's death had anything to do with his army service or not. The postmortem examination showed one tiny area of narrowing in one coronary artery in the heart wall—certainly not enough to shut the vessel off. Why did the man die? We were not very sure in 1942. Today the cause of the man's death seems obvious. The first link in the deadly chain was a life behind the bar with much cigarette smoking, obesity, and no physical conditioning at all; the second link was the appearance of a small amount of hardening in one coronary artery feeding a vital area of heart muscle; and the final link that locked this man to a disaster was the tremendous physical exertion of army basic training. An area of heart muscle suddenly required an enormous increase in blood supply to carry on its work; the extra blood flow could not be supplied through the narrowed coronary artery, and the heart went into a fatal irregularity, probably a ventricular fibrillation. In other words, the heart stopped beating and began a feeble twitching. In minutes the man was dead. The public has seen this kind of episode dramatized on television, heard it over the radio, and read about it in all the popular media. For once the publicity is well deserved and is really quite fortunate. The fact that many of these fatal irregularities can be treated successfully is one of the great advances of modern cardiology.

Fatal arrhythmias may take one of two forms. In **ventricular standstill** (Fig. 5-4, *B*) the ventricles simply stop beating; they lie still as though paralyzed and no blood is pumped at all. The patient drops at once and is dead in minutes unless immediate medical aid is available.

In **ventricular fibrillation** (Fig. 5-4, *A*) the great pumping chambers stop beating and begin a feeble, erratic twitching, which propels no blood at all. The effect is exactly the same as standstill; no blood is pumped, and the patient collapses with death minutes away.

A great number of causes can produce ventricular standstill or ventricular fibrillation. Shock, anesthesia, severe hemorrhage, coronary disease, or sudden, overwhelming, physical load on a diseased heart are all common sources of these disastrous arrhythmias.

Twenty years ago these arrhythmias almost always produced death; in an occasional case a beat might have started spontaneously, but it was exceedingly rare. Then came the first breakthrough; open chest massage was developed. Surgeons found that they could open a chest with an incision between the ribs and

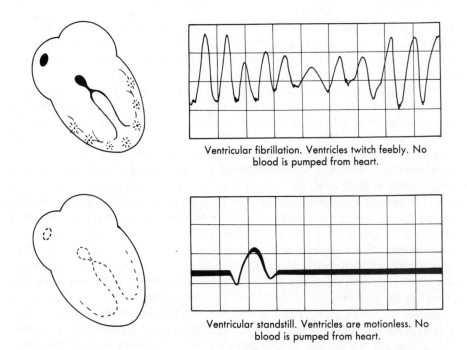

Ventricular fibrillation. Ventricles twitch feebly. No blood is pumped from heart.

Ventricular standstill. Ventricles are motionless. No blood is pumped from heart.

Fig. 5-4. Fatal arrhythmias. Ventricular fibrillation and ventricular standstill. Either of these arrhythmias produces death in a few minutes. No blood is pumped to the brain and cells begin to die in about four minutes. Cardiac massage, artificial respiration, and electric restoration of heartbeat can save the patient's life.

reach in and squeeze the ventricles as one might squeeze a bulb syringe. Blood is squeezed out to the vital organs, just as if the heart were pumping, and life is maintained. Often after a few seconds of this kind of massage the heart begins to beat normally. In other cases drugs and application of electric shock to the heart itself are needed. Many lives are saved, but many still are lost. After all, the ventricles will not always begin to fibrillate in an operating room or in a hospital where a trained surgeon is ready to cut the chest open. Furthermore, the ventricles often refuse to stop fibrillating, even after careful massage by a trained operator.

It goes without saying that somebody must breathe for the patient when the heart stops. When heart massage is being carried on, mouth-to-mouth breathing must be started at once or the whole procedure is useless, of course. The goal of cardiac massage is the delivery of oxygenated blood to the vital tissues of the body, and if the blood isn't oxygenated by breathing, there isn't any point in pumping it around.

About seven years ago workers at Johns Hopkins Medical School found that it is possible to squeeze the heart sufficiently to pump blood by simply pressing down hard on the breastbone. The ventricles are then compressed against the backbone, and blood is pumped out in adequate quantities. This **external massage** can be performed by any trained physician, nurse, attendant, or first-aider. Life can be maintained by external massage and artifical respiration for several hours (Chapter 22).

The last steps in the conquest of these deadly arrhythmias have been electronic. A direct-current shock—the same kind of shock used to end atrial fibrillation—proved to be amazingly effective in halting ventricular fibrillation. Instantaneous shock from a direct-current source is many times safer and more effective than the old alternating-current shock used for years previously. Dr. Lown and his associates at Harvard also contributed to this major advance. The world is considerably in their debt.

In case of standstill that does not respond after massage and administration of drugs, the physician will usually try to drive the heart by an electronic pacemaker. These pacemakers are very much like the electric stimulators used to drive the heart in the presence of complete heart block. A flexible electrode can be threaded into the heart through a vein or pushed through the chest wall by means of a needle. In some cases, the electronic pacemaker will drive the heart very efficiently as long as may be needed; in other types of standstill, especially those associated with very severe coronary disease, the heart may not respond to this kind of pacing. It is always worth a trial and sometimes is spectacularly successful.

Men and women still die of ventricular fibrillation or standstill. However, and this is the triumph, many now live who would have died twenty years ago. The conquest of ventricular fibrillation and standstill, now completed in part, is bringing light into a dark corner of human experience.

6   Coronary artery disease

The term "coronary artery disease" refers to any abnormal condition of the coronary arteries that interferes with the delivery of an adequate supply of blood to the structures of the heart.

Every period of history has had its scourges or plagues. Bubonic plague was the great exterminator during the Middle Ages. Venereal disease decimated and maimed both rich and poor in Renaissance Europe. Pulmonary tuberculosis, high infant mortality, and the whole spectrum of infectious disease were the terrors of the first part of this century. Many of these ogres of the past have vanished, while others have shrunk to easily managed dwarfs.

The role of medicine in the United States and the conquest of many of these diseases has been creditable; one thinks with real pride of the role of American medicine and community action in exterminating so recent a horror as poliomyelitis.

In another area, we—all of us in the Western World—are not doing very well. Somehow, by our own reactions and our own way of life we have created a monster.

Coronary artery disease is the great epidemic disease of the Western World in the twentieth century. It is the "Black Death" of our time. As a cause of cardiac death and disability it is at least ten times as important as any other single affliction of the heart.

Why is coronary artery disease generally rare in the countries of the "Third World," and why does it increase with appalling swiftness whenever one of these countries adopts Western culture and habits? A few years ago coronary artery disease was virtually unknown among the Navajo of Arizona and New Mexico, but with the passage of time and the change of folkways more cases are detected every year. The Soviets describe an increase in death rate throughout the U.S.S.R. due chiefly to the increase in coronary artery disease as more and more previously remote population groups are included in the dubious blessings of Western civilization.

These are fascinating and vital considerations, but before pursuing them it is necessary to explain what coronary disease is and how it affects life and health.

A number of diseases can affect the coronary arteries, but by far the commonest, accounting for over 95% of all coronary artery disease, is a special kind of obstructive degeneration called atherosclerosis or atheromatosis. The words "atheroma" and "atherosclerosis" are going to be used a great deal in the rest of this book, and you should be very clear about their meanings. Imagine that a coronary artery is suddenly enlarged to the size of a garden hose. This gives you a chance to look inside the vessel and in fact to reach into the cut opening and feel the texture of the inside wall. You will find that it is a slick, smooth surface like wet, soft plastic, a surface along which blood could flow swiftly and easily. Now suppose that a wad of putty or chewing gum were stuck to the wall of the hose

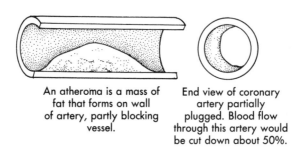

An atheroma is a mass of fat that forms on wall of artery, partly blocking vessel.

End view of coronary artery partially plugged. Blood flow through this artery would be cut down about 50%.

Fig. 6-1. Coronary atheroma. A mass of fatty material growing on the lining of a coronary artery and partially or totally blocking the flow of blood through the vessel.

partially plugging it up; the hose is not completely blocked, and water can still flow through it, but the flow through the area partly plugged with putty or gum will be only about 50% of the water that would come through if the obstruction were not there. This is a good likeness of the formation of an atheroma in the lining of a coronary artery.

An atheroma is a mass of fatty material that forms on the inside wall of a coronary artery, partly or totally plugging, or occluding, the vessel (Fig. 6-1). This fatty mass is made up of all the types of fat, or lipids, that normally circulate in the blood; that is, cholesterol, triglycerides, and phospholipids.

It is important to define several terms carefully at this point. **Sclerosis,** in medical terms, simply means hardening of some tissue or structure. **Arteriosclerosis** is a general term referring to hardening taking place anywhere in the arterial circulation, or tree. **Atherosclerosis** is one particular form of arteriosclerosis that often involves the arteries that carry blood to the heart, brain, kidneys, arms, and legs. It is specifically characterized by the deposits of localized masses of fatty material called atheromas.

The presence of an atheroma on the lining of a coronary artery is bad in itself; worse results follow. Scar tissue, called fibrous tissue, grows into and around the mass of fat, binding it firmly to the arterial wall. Finally, calcium, a hard, chalky material, fills all or part of the mass in the wake of the scar tissue formation. Thus the atheroma, which started as a soft, rubbery mass of fat, ends as a hard, rocklike, chalky plaque resembling a piece of cement stuck to the lining of the artery.

Early or late, fatty or chalky, an atheroma may grow to such a size that it blocks the coronary artery very significantly or even completely like a boulder damming a stream.

A blood clot is very likely to form anyplace in a blood vessel where the blood is partly "dammed up." This often happens immediately "upstream" from an atheroma (Fig. 6-2, *D*). Once the blood clot has formed, it extends down and sometimes past the original atheroma. The medical term for a blood clot is a **thrombus.** When a thrombus forms in the coronary artery, the condition is called coronary thrombosis, meaning stoppage of a coronary artery by a blood clot.

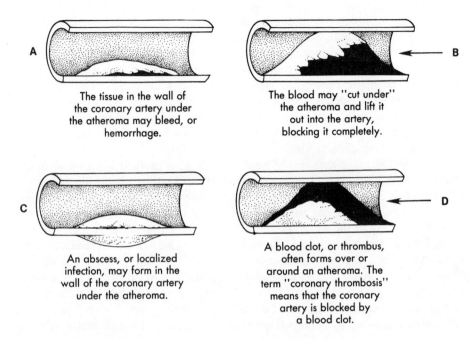

A, The tissue in the wall of
the coronary artery under
the atheroma may bleed, or
hemorrhage.

B, The blood may "cut under"
the atheroma and lift it
out into the artery,
blocking it completely.

C, An abscess, or localized
infection, may form in the
wall of the coronary artery
under the atheroma.

D, A blood clot, or thrombus,
often forms over or
around an atheroma. The
term "coronary thrombosis"
means that the coronary
artery is blocked by
a blood clot.

Fig. 6-2. Complications of coronary atheroma. **A,** The tissue in the wall of the coronary artery under the atheroma may bleed, or hemorrhage. **B,** The blood may "cut under" the atheroma and lift it out into the artery, blocking it completely. **C,** An abscess, or localized infection, may form in the wall of the coronary artery under the atheroma. **D,** A blood clot, or thrombus, often forms over or around an atheroma. The term *coronary thrombosis* means that the coronary artery is blocked by a blood clot.

Blood clots in the coronary arteries practically always form around a diseased area, usually an atheroma. Sometimes there will be bleeding of the tissue immediately under the atheroma. The bleeding tends to separate the plaque from the wall of the blood vessel as if it had been dissected off with a knife. The plaque then lifts out into the bloodstream and fall across the artery, blocking it completely (Fig. 6-2, *B*). Finally, infection or death of tissue under the atheroma may form an abscess in the wall of the artery immediately under the plaque. This will have the same effect as hemorrhage; the plaque will again "lift off" and block the artery completely (Fig. 6-2, *C*).

CLINICAL MANIFESTATIONS OF CORONARY ARTERY DISEASE

The human race first became aware of the effects of coronary atheromatosis in the eighteenth century when an English physician named Heberden wrote a description of an illness he called "angina pectoris." The victims of this affliction, he noted, felt a smothering sensation in the breast, which often was so alarming that the patient feared death; this discomfort was brought on by physical effort, such as climbing a hill, ascending stairs, or performing manual labor. It was promptly relieved by rest.

It is a tribute to the human intellect that in 1786 without benefit of instruments, depending solely on reason and intuition, Heberden postulated that this set of symptoms was connected with the heart; his idea was confirmed when his great colleague, Jenner (discoverer of smallpox vaccine) performed an autopsy on a victim of the angina pectoris at Bath and noted "a white, fleshy protuberance in the lumen of the coronary artery." He wondered in a letter to Heberden if this obstructing mass might not be the cause of the discomfort brought on by exertion and relieved by rest. It was the first causal connection between coronary atheromatosis and clinical disease.

Both Heberden and Jenner were right. Angina pectoris is the result of obstructive disease of one or more coronary arteries; it is the classic and commonest manifestation of the disease. Fig. 6-3 illustrates the mechanism of angina pectoris.

Briefly, a narrowing in a coronary artery cuts down the blood flow to a critical point; thus the heart muscle depending on that blood vessel has just enough blood for its needs when the heart is beating slowly, doing relatively little work. The heart responds to any exertion by beating faster, of course; when it beats faster it needs more oxygen—that is, blood. The narrowing in the diseased coronary artery does not permit the necessary increase in blood flow to compensate for the effects of exercise, and so an area of heart muscle does not receive an adequate oxygen supply. The patient often notes some kind of discomfort when

---

Fig. 6-3. Mechanism of angina pectoris. **A,** A diver depends on his hose for air. He has no other source. **B,** Similarly, an area of heart muscle depends on a branch of a coronary artery for blood. It has no other source. **C,** The diver's hose is kinked. There is still enough air if he sits quietly and does not breathe hard. **D,** A coronary artery is partly blocked by an atheroma. Blood flow is cut in half. There is still enough blood for the needs of the heart muscle if the heart does not work very hard. **E,** If the diver must struggle violently, he will have to breathe hard, since his body needs more oxygen. The kinked air hose limits his supply of air. He begins to feel suffocated and tugs on the air hose to warn those on the surface of his trouble. **F,** The patient climbs stairs, walks up a hill, or eats a big meal. His heart is forced to beat faster and work harder, and the heart muscle needs more blood for his extra work. The heart muscle depends upon a narrowed, diseased coronary artery for its blood supply. It will not receive the extra blood it needs for the extra work load. The patient will usually feel pain or some other type of discomfort. It is the body's way of telling him that some area of heart muscle is not receiving enough blood. **G,** The oxygen supply falls below the danger point. The diver falls into a coma. He is in danger of dying, but he is not dead yet. If the hose unkinks and he receives more oxygen, he can still recover. **H,** Blood flow to an area of heart muscle falls below the amount needed to keep the cells alive. The cells are damaged, but they are not dead yet. If the blood flow increases, the cells can still recover. They can also recover if they need less blood, that is, if the heart is put at rest. **I,** The diver's oxygen supply is completely cut off. He dies. **J,** Blood flow to an area of heart muscle is completely cut off. The heart muscle dies. When tissue in any part of the body dies because its supply is cut off through blocking or hemorrhage of a terminal artery, the dead area is called an infarct.

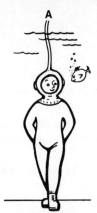

A

A diver depends on his hose for air. He has no other source.

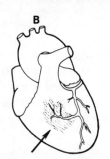

B

Similarly, an area of heart muscle depends on a branch of a coronary artery for blood. It has no other source.

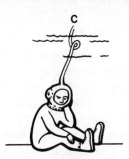

C

The diver's hose is kinked. There is still enough air if he sits quietly and doesn't breathe hard.

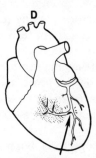

D

A coronary artery is partly blocked by an atheroma. Blood flow is cut in half. There is still enough blood for the needs of the heart muscle if the heart doesn't work very hard.

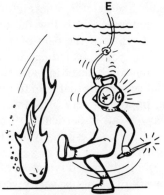

E

If the diver must struggle violently, he will have to breathe hard, since his body needs more oxygen. The kinked air hose limits his supply of air. He begins to feel suffocated, and tugs on the air hose to warn those on the surface of his trouble.

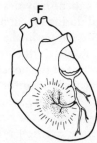

F

The patient climbs stairs, walks up a hill, or eats a big meal. His heart is forced to beat faster and work harder, and the heart muscle needs more blood for his extra work. The heart muscle depends upon a narrowed, diseased coronary artery for its blood supply. It will not receive the extra blood it needs for the extra work load. The patient will usually feel pain or some other type of discomfort. It is the body's way of telling him that some area of heart muscle is not receiving enough blood.

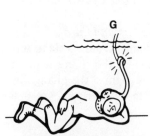

G

The oxygen supply falls below the danger point. The diver falls into a coma. He is in danger of dying, but he is not dead yet. If the hose unkinks and he receives more oxygen, he can still recover.

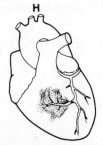

H

Blood flow to an area of heart muscle falls below the amount needed to keep the cells alive. The cells are damaged, but they are not dead yet. If the blood flow increases, the cells can still recover. They can also recover if they need less blood, that is, if the heart is put at rest.

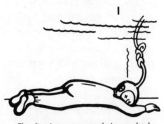

I

The diver's oxygen supply is completely cut off. He dies.

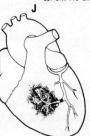

J

Blood flow to an area of heart muscle is completely cut off. The heart muscle dies. When tissue in any part of the body dies because its supply is cut off through blocking or hemorrhage of a terminal artery, the dead area is called an infarct.

this happens. The discomfort tends to disappear when the exertion is halted because the heartrate falls and the needs of the heart muscle can now be met by the
subnormal flow rate through the diseased artery.

*"Classic" angina pectoris, therefore, is discomfort produced by exertion
and relieved by rest; it is caused by narrowing of one or more coronary arteries,
almost always by atheromatosis.*

Any activity that increases the heart rate, raises the blood pressure, or
both will increase the oxygen requirements of the heart muscle and may thus be
the trigger for an attack of angina pectoris. The symptoms cover a wide range.
The patient may describe them as a sensation of pressure under the breastbone
noted during exertion, possibly a sense of tightness into the shoulder and the jaw,
or discomfort in the upper abdomen just below the breastbone, in either arm,
and, rarely, in the upper back. In fact, the pain of angina pectoris may be felt
anywhere in the upper half of the torso, including the ears; the consistent feature
is that the discomfort is brought on by exertion and relieved by rest.

There are some special conditions that help to precipitate angina pectoris.
A large meal, for example, imposes a very heavy workload on the heart, and
therefore exertion after heavy meals is particularly likely to trigger an attack.
Again, exertion performed in the cold especially when walking against a cold
wind commonly initiates an attack.

Pain is the most commonly described symptom of angina pectoris, but it is
not the only one; the victim will often notice very severe shortness of breath accompanied by apprehension, a sensation of pounding of the heart, or sometimes
mild perspiration. In all forms of classic, or typical, angina the sequence of exertion—discomfort—rest—relief will be consistent and will alert the physician to
the possibility of angina pectoris and the underlying coronary artery disease that
produces it.

*Typical effort-related angina pectoris will appear in one of two quite dif-
ferent forms—stable or unstable.*

*Every patient with coronary artery disease must understand the distinction
between these two forms of the syndrome* because the change from stable to unstable angina pectoris is a medical crisis. Failure to recognize the change can be
fatal, and it is the patient, after all, who will have to recognize the change in
symptoms that conveys the only warning of an impending disaster.

Stable angina pectoris

Stable angina pectoris is angina that is predictably brought on by the same
level of effort. For example, a patient with stable angina pectoris will note that it
is possible to walk three blocks briskly before pain appears or may find that it is
possible to climb a certain set of stairs or play a certain number of games of tennis
without producing discomfort. The experienced patient can predict with surprising accuracy the kind of exertion that will produce discomfort and what can be
safely tolerated. Stable angina pectoris is a condition millions of people live with
while they carry on their normal gainful activities, pursue reasonable recreation,
and often live out a normal life expectancy.

Unstable angina pectoris

Unstable angina pectoris, on the other hand, is never benign; it is always dangerous and it always demands immediate treatment. When a physician diagnoses unstable angina, the disease has become progressively more severe in one of several ways.

1. The angina begins to appear with lower levels of effort; the patient who could walk three blocks comfortably, for example, now feels pain after walking only one.
2. The pain becomes more severe. The patient who found that angina could be controlled with one tablet of nitroglycerin now must take three or four, and even this may not be enough.
3. The pain appears more frequently and now is sometimes not provoked by exercise but rather appears even when the patient is resting quietly.

This increase in severity can be abrupt or gradual. When the unstable, or **crescendo,** effect comes on slowly, it may not be easy to detect at first, but both patient and physician must be alert to this kind of change in the quality of the disease.

Unstable angina pectoris is a medical crisis; it calls for immediate hospitalization in an intensive care unit. If the syndrome is recognized and appropriate therapy is begun, the risk is very small; if it goes unnoticed and untreated, the risk of myocardial infarction and sudden death is high.

Prinzmetal angina

Myron Prinzmetal in the 1930's described a kind of angina that is completely different from the distress described so eloquently 200 years before by Dr. Heberden. With the kind of angina Prinzmetal described the victim notices the pain *without* any relation to exertion; it simply comes on abruptly, possibly when the patient is sitting quietly, working, or performing minimal activity. The quality of the discomfort is exactly the same as in effort-related exertion. Prinzmetal angina is often noted at night; it will characteristically awaken the patient in the early morning hours with a feeling of discomfort of some kind, often accompanied by "smothering" and severe apprehension.

Prinzmetal, or variant, angina is sometimes associated with severe atheromatous disease at the beginning, or origin, of one of the three major coronary arteries. Sometimes it appears in patients who have anatomically normal coronary arteries. There are no atheromas in them; the problem in these patients is that the artery goes into *spasm,* that is, contracts itself violently, like a fist closing, enough to turn off the flow of blood to the heart muscle and produce symptoms.

To the concept of coronary atheromas blocking the flow of blood, you must now add a second concept, that is, the concept of spasm, or contraction, of the artery, doing the same thing. Both arteries and veins have coats of muscle, and either an artery or a vein under the right conditions can contract so forcefully that the flow of blood is seriously diminished or even shut off entirely.

Myocardial infarction—"heart attack"

The word "infarct" is a medical term referring to an area of tissue that dies because its blood supply has been cut off. Infarcts, or dead areas, may form in the brain, the kidneys, the liver, or in many other areas of the body, but they are most common and probably most dangerous in the wall of the heart.

A coronary atheroma may grow so large that it simply stops the vessel completely, producing a myocardial infarct; hemorrhage, abscess, or blood clot forming in an atheromatous area may do the same thing. For any of these reasons (and the medical profession really isn't sure which is "the chicken" and which is "the egg" in many cases) the atheromatous vessel finally is completely stopped up, and the tissue that depends on that vessel for its vital nutrients begins to die.

Collateral coronary circulation is a key phenomenon to keep in mind at this point; the problem is that in many patients it isn't very good. Most organs and tissues of the body have a double and sometimes a triple blood supply. Each finger, for example, has an artery running up each side with many cross-connections, or collaterals (Fig. 6-4). If one artery to a finger were stopped up, the finger would not be lost; blood would flow through the collateral circulation from the other artery, and the needs of the cells in the finger would be met.

The coronary arteries have the poorest set of collateral connections in the body. In many patients these vessels simply end without any cross-connections to other vessels, thus a given area of heart muscle will depend on one particular branch of a coronary artery for its blood supply, and if that branch is stopped up, the area of muscle will die. Everything else being equal, a patient with many collateral cross-connections of the coronary arteries is more likely to survive a coronary occlusion than one with poor collaterals.

A myocardial infarct is usually a very sudden event, although it may be preceded by a period of unstable, or crescendo, angina.

When heart muscle is infarcted, a certain amount of heart muscle is always totally lost—that is, it ends up as dead scar tissue, not capable of performing the normal contracting motions of heart muscle. The seriousness of the myocardial infarct is in direct proportion to the amount of muscle lost, and this is a matter of chance because the amount of muscle lost depends on how high up in the arterial tree the blockage occurs and how good the collateral vessels are to the infarcted area. If the area of dead muscle is small, say in the range of the size of a pea or a dime, the risk is probably not very great. On the other hand, if the infarcted area involves 30% to 40% of the total left ventricular mass, the patient is almost certainly going to die.

Once the blood supply to the heart muscle has been cut off and the infarct has formed, it takes a certain minimum amount of time for the tissue to die and to heal with strong scar formation (Fig. 6-5). The total healing process is in the range of six to eight weeks, never less. After the first forty-eight hours the tissue in the infarct may look reddish or purple and have a hard consistency, something like the tissue around the edge of a very large boil. After about ten to fourteen days the tissue that has no blood supply at all has actually died, leaving a soft, dark center that looks something like a thumbnail that has been smashed by a

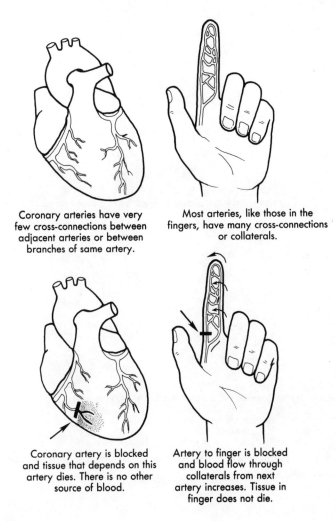

Coronary arteries have very few cross-connections between adjacent arteries or between branches of same artery.

Most arteries, like those in the fingers, have many cross-connections or collaterals.

Coronary artery is blocked and tissue that depends on this artery dies. There is no other source of blood.

Artery to finger is blocked and blood flow through collaterals from next artery increases. Tissue in finger does not die.

Fig. 6-4. Collateral circulation. Structural weakness of the coronary arteries.

hammer. Around the edge of this area there will be some tissue that did not lose its blood supply completely and is in the process of healing. After six to eight weeks a hard, white scar will have formed in the wall of the heart.

The risk of myocardial infarction

The initial risk of death with myocardial infarction is very high; about 50% of the victims die before they reach a hospital or receive other medical attention. Once a patient reaches a hospital where adequate medical care is available, the risk is much smaller—in the range of 10% to 15% overall.

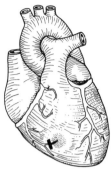

First day—vessel completely blocked; heart muscle injured.

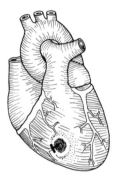

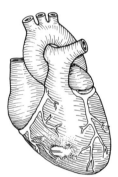

Tenth day—central area of dead
heart muscle (black); zone of
injured, but still living, muscle
surrounds it.

6 to 8 weeks—
scar forming
in heart wall.

Fig. 6-5. Evolution of a myocardial infarct. Progressive changes in heart muscle following stoppage of a coronary artery.

Complications of myocardial infarction; causes of death

It is an odd fact of medical history that even though the significance of coronary disease has been known for over a century and a half, nobody knew exactly what a myocardial infarct was until Dr. Herrick defined the process in his history-making studies in Chicago in 1912. Older generations might remember all sorts of fanciful reasons for sudden death such as "acute indigestion," "heart seizures," and the like. For decades after the discovery of the true nature of myocardial infarction physicians knew that infarction often was followed by sudden death, but not until the last twenty years has the medical profession really learned how and why this happens.

Cardiac arrhythmias. One of the two fatal cardiac arrhythmias (Chapter 5), ventricular fibrillation, or ventricular standstill, is practically always the cause of sudden death at the time of the infarct. Even among patients who survive to reach a coronary care unit in a hospital the risk of fatal arrhythmias persists. This risk is highest in the first few hours after the infarct, but it is still significant for three to five days, depending on the severity of the infarct and its location. Specialized coronary care units were originally organized primarily to deal with these life-threatening arrhythmias.

Heart block. Failure of conduction from atria to ventricles of various types and degrees may appear in the course of the evolution of the infarct. Some types of block are relatively harmless, while others urgently require the insertion of a pacemaker. This is another reason that the patient needs to be in a specialized coronary care unit where the electrocardiogram can be observed continuously on an oscilloscope.

Shock. The term "shock" has a precise medical definition; it is important to differentiate it from the loose application of the word in describing horror, surprise, or some other sudden, unpleasant state of mind. True physical **shock** is an abnormal state of the body that results when there is an inadequate volume of circulating blood. This can happen for a number of reasons—blood loss from a wound, crushing injury, and overwhelming infections among others, but the common denominator is that there is not enough blood to bring adequate flow to the vital organs of the body. As a result of the low blood volume the blood pressure falls, the pulse becomes rapid and weak as the heart tries to beat rapidly to make up for the inadequate volume, the brain slows its functions because of lack of blood flow, the patient becomes confused or even loses consciousness, and the kidneys stop manufacturing adequate amounts of urine because they are not receiving enough blood to perform their normal filtering function.

Myocardial infarction is sometimes followed by shock; it is an extremely serious complication with a high death rate and calls for skilled medical intervention.

Congestive heart failure (Chapter 3). The great majority of all infarcts take place in the left ventricle, either in the free wall or in the intraventricular septum. Naturally there is some loss of pumping efficiency when muscle is injured or dead; when a critical amount of muscle is thus taken out of function, congestive heart failure may follow because the damaged ventricle simply cannot pump the blood out of the lungs as fast as the right ventricle is pumping it *in.* Congestive failure may appear hours or days following the actual myocardial infarct as the effect of the tissue death slowly manifests itself. Most myocardial infarcts will produce some degree of myocardial failure, but in the great majority of cases it will be mild, requiring nothing more than diuretics and occasionally digitalis. When severe congestive heart failure appears soon after myocardial infarction, however, it implies that a significant amount of tissue has been destroyed in the left ventricle and the outlook becomes much more serious. The physician will often have to use specialized equipment to record pressures inside the heart and in the arteries and will have to manipulate the balance of fluid load and pressures on the heart very carefully. Severe congestive heart failure can be successfully treated, but it will often call for specialized equipment and highly trained personnel.

• • •

Any of these complications are likely to appear in the early stages of myocardial infarction. The patient must therefore be observed carefully, preferably in an intensive cardiac care unit. Many of these specialized units are now in opera-

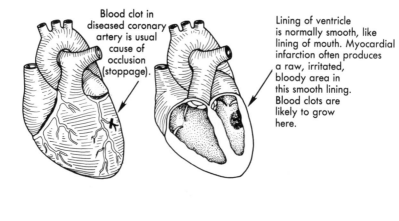

Blood clot in diseased coronary artery is usual cause of occlusion (stoppage).

Lining of ventricle is normally smooth, like lining of mouth. Myocardial infarction often produces a raw, irritated, bloody area in this smooth lining. Blood clots are likely to grow here.

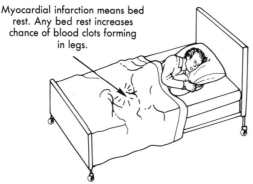

Myocardial infarction means bed rest. Any bed rest increases chance of blood clots forming in legs.

Fig. 6-6. Blood clots as a complication of myocardial infarction.

tion, and it is hoped that within the very near future every hospital will be so equipped. In an intensive coronary care unit physicians, nurses, and trained aides will carry out intensive care during the high-risk period following an acute coronary thrombosis with myocardial infarction. This critical period, in which the patient must be carefully supervised, covers at least four days after the coronary occlusion; it often extends to seven days.

No patient with myocardial infarction can be said to be free of complications until at least two and preferably three weeks have passed.

Coronary insufficiency, or intermediate coronary syndrome

The intermediate coronary syndrome is a kind of halfway house between unstable angina pectoris and true myocardial infarction. In simple angina pectoris the cells are for a short time receiving an inadequate blood supply, but when the needs of the heart muscle are reduced so that the period of "short supply" is over, the cells return to normal function. There is no permanent damage. In myocardial infarction the cells undergo permanent, irreversible change and often end as white, inert scar tissue. In coronary insufficiency, or intermediate coronary syndrome, the situation is somewhere between the two. The blood supply to the cells is cut down for a longer period than with simple angina pectoris, and they actually undergo some degenerative changes. By definition the pain of an intermediate coronary syndrome lasts thirty minutes or more and is not immediately relieved by simply stopping activity or taking the appropriate medicine. The electrocardiogram undergoes progressive changes, although they are not the typical changes of myocardial infarction.

The distinction between an intermediate coronary syndrome and a true myocardial infarct is one that can only be made by careful laboratory and electrocardiographic studies. Symptoms may be identical, and the patient will need to be hospitalized until the physician can decide which of the two conditions is present.

DIAGNOSIS OF CORONARY ARTERY DISEASE

How can a patient tell that coronary disease is actually present? How is it possible to distinguish between the various clinical syndromes and with what degree of accuracy? Is there any way to estimate the risk the patient faces, both immediate and long term? How can the patient be advised intelligently about safe limits at work, physical activity, and life-style and, above all, about the type of therapy needed for the disease?

Diagnosis in coronary artery disease rests on one or more of six basic elements:

1. History. Any experienced physician relies on the patient's own description of his illness for three quarters of most diagnoses. (The history of the illness, that is, the detailed story of the way the symptoms appeared, what they felt like, what part of the body they involved, what made them worse and what relieved them, is more important than any instruments or gadgets ever invented.)

The value of a careful history has been stressed; be patient when your physician asks a great many questions. Careful history-taking is the mark of a skilled clinician.

Sometimes the simplest inquiry will be decisive; for example, coronary artery disease is very rare in people under 30 and relatively rare in those under 40. It is also extremely rare in females before menopause. Thus when a 30-year-old female describes chest pain, the astute clinician will look for other causes than coronary disease. The pain of ischemic heart muscle is never influenced by breathing. When a patient describes pain in the chest that is caused only by breathing, disappearing when the breath is held, it is clear without further study that the pain does not originate in the heart muscle. True angina pectoris is produced by exertion that causes a rise in pulse rate, systolic blood pressure, or both; it is not produced or made worse by simple motions of the arm or shoulder. When a patient can reproduce pain in the upper left chest by moving the arm about or by pushing on the ribs, that pain is clearly arising from the muscles and tendons of the region not from the heart.

2. Physical examination. The physical examination with stethoscope and fingertips may be completely normal, even in the presence of severe coronary ar-

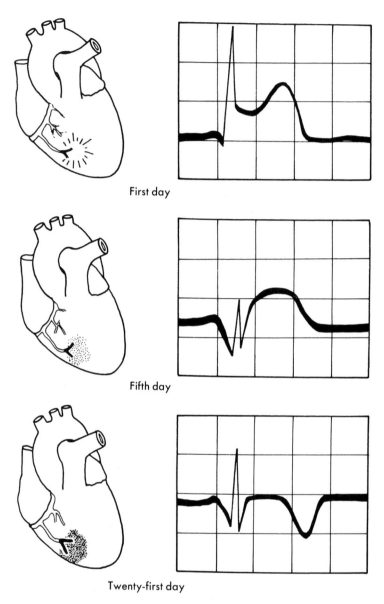

First day

Fifth day

Twenty-first day

Fig. 6-7. Progressive change in the electrocardiogram during the evolution of a myocardial infarction.

tery disease. Abnormal physical findings will often be helpful, however, in detecting complications such as early heart failure or abnormalities of heartwall motion due to scarring, arrhythmias, etc.

3. Electrocardiogram. The resting electrocardiogram is a cornerstone of

modern cardiac diagnosis; it should always be recorded as part of the initial evaluation of any patient suspected of having coronary artery disease. There are specific progressive electrocardiographic changes in the presence of myocardial infarction and intermediate coronary syndrome (Fig. 6-7).

The resting electrocardiogram may be completely normal, even in the presence of severe symptomatic coronary artery disease; for this reason the exercise electrocardiogram, or stress test, has been evolved to improve the sensitivity of the method by recording a tracing during symptoms or at peak effort. The exercise electrocardiogram will be discussed on the following pages.

4. X-ray results. The routine chest x-ray examination of the heart and lungs is of sporadic value. The x-ray results are often totally normal in the presence of severe coronary artery disease, but they may be helpful in detecting calcified atheromas in the coronary arteries. (The calcium will appear as small, white lines on the x-ray film, and this finding correlates to a remarkable degree with severe coronary artery disease.) The chest x-ray examination also will be invaluable in detecting cardiac enlargement and congestive heart failure.

5. Cardiac enzymes. The blood enzymes referred to are complex chemicals contained in heart muscle cells. When these cells begin to die as a result of infarction, the enzymes are released into the blood and can be detected very accurately. The presence or absence of these markers of dead heart muscle may be crucial in the diagnosis of myocardial infarction; the value of this determination is universally accepted.

6. Coronary arteriography. The technique of coronary arteriography involves introducing a catheter into an artery in the arm or the groin, passing it up the aorta to the actual orifice, or mouth, of the coronary arteries, and injecting dye into the vessel while recording x-ray "motion pictures," or cineangiograms, which show the passage of the dye through the vessels with remarkable clarity and fidelity (Fig. 6-8). The coronary arteriogram is not totally accurate because there are sources of error as in any test, but the method certainly must be considered the final yardstick for demonstrating abnormalities of the coronary arteries against which all other methods can be evaluated. In other words, coronary arteriography is the best method available today for demonstrating both anatomy and disease of the coronary arteries. It will be discussed further on pp. 63 to 65.

Exercise electrocardiogram, or treadmill exercise testing, and coronary arteriography are the two "high-technology" techniques evolved in the past twenty years. Practically every patient with coronary artery disease will be asked to consider undergoing one or both of these tests. The usefulness, limitations, and risks of each will be described in sufficient detail to help the patient make an informed judgment about the need for the tests and the evaluation of the results.

Exercise electrocardiogram

The resting electrocardiogram may be completely normal in a patient with coronary disease. Sometimes it will be abnormal, but there is no specific pattern of abnormality associated with angina pectoris as such.

During an attack of angina, however, there will practically always be a change in the electrocardiogram. An injury current will be generated by the heart

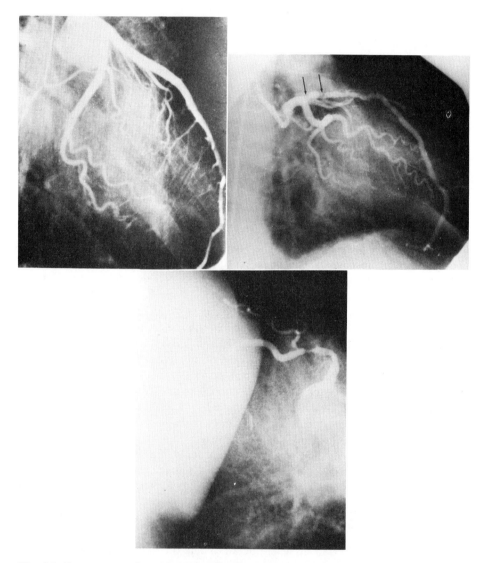

Fig. 6-8. Coronary arteriography. Visualization of the coronary arteries by injection of dye through a catheter. (Courtesy of Gordon Ewy, M.D., University of Arizona.)

Resting (normal) ECG

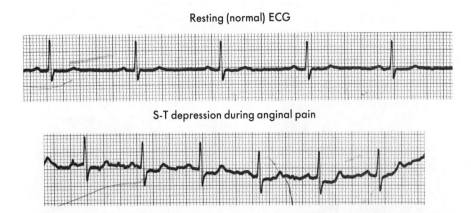

S-T depression during anginal pain

Fig. 6-9. ST depression on the electrocardiogram, representing an injury current detected during an attack of angina pectoris.

muscle, which is at that moment undersupplied with blood, and this "injury current" will record as an upward or downward movement of the "quiet interval" of the electrocardiogram—the ST segment, or the period immediately after the end of ventricular activation (Fig. 6-9). Obviously, a physician couldn't follow a patient around all day trundling an electrocardiograph, waiting for an attack of angina pectoris; various means have been evolved to produce angina under controlled conditions in the heart laboratory where the electrocardiogram can be observed during and after the attack. The earliest method was evolved by Dr. Arthur Master and simply consisted of having the patient mount a given set of small stairs a given number of times until pain was produced and then quickly recording the electrocardiogram. More sophisticated techniques have evolved, and now every heart laboratory in the world is equipped with some kind of exercise machine for the purpose of inducing angina or its equivalent.

Most commonly a treadmill is used (Fig. 6-10). A number of electrodes are attached to the patient so that the standard electrocardiographic leads can be recorded throughout exercise. These are usually viewed on an oscilloscope and a permanent record is made on a standard multiple-channel electrocardiograph. The speed of the treadmill and the elevation against which the patient walks is increased every three minutes according to one of several standard patterns so that a carefully calculated increase in oxygen need is generated. It takes about three minutes at each increased stage of exercise for the body to accommodate: that is, for the heart rate to increase, for the stroke volume to rise, and for the body to begin extracting more oxygen from each unit of blood flowing through the lungs. Because the progression in exercise is carefully graded, these are referred to as "graded exercise tolerance tests."

The exercise is continued to one of three end points:

1. The patient notices the appearance of discomfort characteristic of angina.

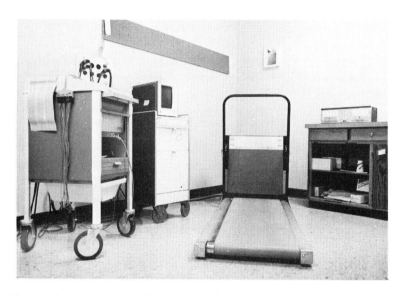

Fig. 6-10. Exercise-treadmill lab. Pictured is equipment commonly used in exercise testing for coronary disease including (left to right) a 3-channel electrocardiograph oscilloscope, treadmill, and defibrillating equipment.

2. An injury current is recorded on the ST segment of the electrocardiogram.
3. One of several danger signs is noted that causes the physician to halt the test—a falling blood pressure, a sense of extreme shortness of breath and apprehension on the part of the patient, or one of several types of arrhythmia.

The electrocardiogram is observed for five to ten minutes in the postexercise state, and if the cardiologist is thorough, the patient will be examined with a stethoscope for abnormal heart sounds in the postexercise period.

The cardiologist will grade the results of the test in one of several ways:

1. ST segment change. The cardiologist will want to see not only *how much* the ST segments are elevated or depressed, but also what their shape is. Normal people will show depression of the beginning of this important segment with exercise, but it will be what is called "junction" depression, meaning that the segment slopes sharply up from this initial point of depression. This is a normal variant and does not imply the presence of disease. On the other hand, if the entire ST segment is depressed and "flat" for at least 0.08 seconds (two of the small squares on the electrocardiogram paper) or if the ST segment is depressed and then slopes downward for the rest of its course, the finding becomes significant (Fig. 6-11).

The more the ST segments move (up or down), the more likely it is that the change in the electrocardiogram is really a consequence of underperfusion of heart muscle. Thus if the ST segments in one or more leads were only slightly de-

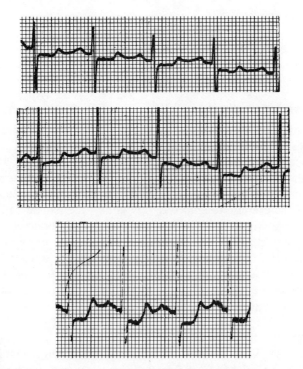

Fig. 6-11. Types of ST change produced during treadmill exercises. The deeper the ST depression, the more significant the change.

pressed (for instance, 0.5 millimeters) without other findings, the cardiologist should be very cautious about assuming the presence of coronary artery disease. If they were depressed 1 millimeter, he could be more confident, and if they were depressed 1.5 to 2 millimeters, the accuracy of the test would be very high.

2. Anginal pain. If a patient feels typical anginal distress during exertion and if this distress is relieved by rest, the cardiologist has significant evidence for the presence of coronary artery disease. If this typical anginal distress is accompanied by an "ischemic" ST depression (the flatter, down-sloping type described earlier), the accuracy of the test rises even more. If anginal distress produced on the treadmill is accompanied by 2 millimeters or greater depression of the ST segments, the accuracy of the test is close to 100%. It is also likely that several coronary arteries are severely involved.

3. Anginal equivalents. Sometimes the victim of coronary artery disease will notice other sensations besides pain on exertion. Very severe shortness of breath, apprehension, and sweating will all be signals to the experienced cardiologist to halt the test, whether changes appear on the electrocardiogram or not.

4. Blood pressure response. Normally the systolic, or top, blood pressure rises as the pulse rate goes up during exercise and falls as it returns to baseline. If, however, the blood pressure actually drops during exercise, it it likely that very

severe, widespread coronary artery disease is present and that the heart is simply not capable of generating an adequate response in terms of volume of blood pumped. Sometimes a falling blood pressure will be the consequence of emotional tension or other secondary factors, but as a rule a falling blood pressure with exertion indicates grave cardiac impairment.

"Staging" of the disease

Treadmill testing can also give the cardiologist some idea of just how severe the disease is as well as whether it is present or not. If a patient feels pain or shows electrocardiographic change or other abnormality at a very low level of exertion, the implication is clear that the disease in the coronary arteries must be severe and must potentially threaten a significant area of heart muscle. On the other hand, if the exercise tolerance is very good—the patient can exercise very strenuously before symptoms appear or the electrocardiogram changes—the implication is equally clear that the disease is mild and may very well be something that the patient can live with with some adjustment in life-style and with medical management. The possibility of analyzing coronary disease quantitatively, that is, judging how severe it is as well as determining whether it is present or not is a very important function of treadmill testing.

False-positive and false-negative results

The exercise tolerance test is not infallible! There will always be both false-positive and false-negative tests. A **false-positive** test means that a patient *without* coronary artery disease manifests what are apparently significant electrocardiographic changes during stress testing. Nobody knows why this disturbing response appears in normal patients; it seems to be commoner in middle-aged women than in others, but it can be seen in either sex, most commonly in the group over 40. The percentage of false-positive responses in any large series of studies will run at least 15% of all persons tested and sometimes will be much higher, depending on the kind of group being studied.

False-negative tests are also a problem. As many as 25% of patients with documented coronary artery disease may have a completely normal exercise tolerance test. Partly this is because the exercise test measures function, not anatomy. There may be narrowing in one or more coronary arteries, but this narrowing may not be severe enough to drop the blood supply to the particular region of heart muscle below the danger point, even during strenuous exercise. Thus the exercise test records only the balance or imbalance between supply of blood and demand of the heart muscle during increasing effort; it does not give a precise picture of the structural abnormality within the coronary arteries.

• • •

By combining observations about the kind of discomfort produced, the stage of exercise at which it is produced, the depth of ST depression and the number of electrocardiographic leads in which that depression is noted, the blood pressure change, and the physical examination, the experienced cardiologist can increase the accuracy of the tests greatly, but both patient and physician should always keep in mind that there is substantial room for error.

Coronary arteriography

Coronary arteriography is one of the great technical advances in diagnostic cardiology of all time. With this technique it is possible for the cardiologist to actually see the coronary arteries in great and precise detail.

To record a coronary arteriogram, a thin, flexible, hollow tube called a catheter is introduced into an artery of the arm or leg and threaded up the vessel toward the heart under fluoroscopic guidance. When the tip of the catheter reaches the base of the aorta, where the coronary arteries originate, it is actually maneuvered into the opening of the left and right coronary arteries in turn, and a quantity of opaque dye, which makes a white shadow on x-ray film, is injected into the vessel. X-ray movies, or cineangiograms, are recorded during the procedure (Fig. 6-8, *A* and *B*). Before going further, you should turn to Fig. 6-12 and become familiar with the anatomy of the coronary arteries. The left and right coronary arteries open almost across from each other at the root of the aorta, just beyond the point where that vessel leads out of the left ventricle. The left coronary artery quickly divides into two branches, one running down the front of the heart and one circling around behind it. The main left coronary artery before branching is referred to as the left main coronary artery (LMCA). The branch going down the front of the heart is called the left anterior descending (LAD) coronary artery. The branch curling around behind is called the left circumflex artery (LCA). The right coronary artery descends toward the bottom surface of the heart, the part resting on the diaphragm, and also sends branches to the posterior, or back, wall and throughout a great deal of the "middle" part of the heart.

There are thus four principal coronary arteries; every patient with coronary artery disease should be familiar with them. These are (1) the left main coronary artery (LMCA), (2) the left anterior descending (LAD) coronary artery, (3) the left circumflex artery (LCA), (4) the right coronary artery (RCA).

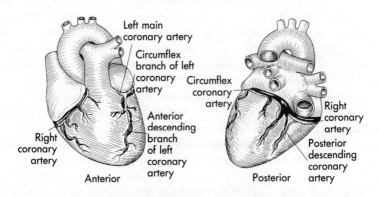

Fig. 6-12. Detailed anatomy of the coronary arteries.

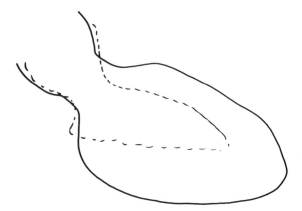

Fig. 6-13. Ventriculogram. Outline of the ventricle in systole and diastole determined during cardiac catheterization. This permits a measurement of the efficiency of ventricular pumping function.

Visualization of the coronary arteries is only one of the observations made when the heart is catheterized. After the coronary artery injection is completed, the cardiologist will thread the catheter on through the aortic valve into the left ventricular cavity. A sufficient quantity of dye is injected to fill the left ventricle, and the cardiologist can now actually see and record quantitatively the pumping action of the heart (Fig. 6-13). By measuring the difference in the inside diameter of the left ventricle in dilation, or diastole, and in contraction, or systole, in several different views, it is possible to calculate the efficiency of the ventricle in ejecting blood. This figure is called the *ejection fraction.* This is the most sensitive measurement available of ventricular function. By watching the cineangiograms through a number of heart cycles, the cardiologist can see the motion of the muscular wall of the ventricle and can detect abnormal motion characteristic of scarred or weakened muscle.

Therefore a complete **cardiac catheterization** for the study of coronary artery disease will include adequate views of all coronary arteries and a well-defined **ventriculogram,** permitting evaluation of left ventricular function.

Coronary arteriography is a giant stride in cardiac diagnosis; the technique permits the cardiologist to detect precisely which coronary artery is diseased and to what extent, while the left ventriculogram gives the most accurate picture of left ventricular function available by modern techniques. However, like everything in human affairs there are minuses and pluses in this equation. Even with a remarkable technique like coronary arteriography, there is still room for error. Qualified cardiologists often disagree over precise interpretation of films, and for technical reasons significant lesions within the coronary arteries may be missed entirely.

Catheterization of the left side of the heart carries a significant risk to life and health. Simply placing a catheter tip in the opening of a coronary artery creates a certain mechanical obstruction; when the artery is filled with dye instead of blood, the delivery of oxygen to the heart muscle is drastically reduced for a few seconds. Brief bursts of ventricular fibrillation are common at this time, but they can usually be ended quickly without significant harm. Sometimes, however, the heart will go into irreversible ventricular fibrillation, and the patient will die. Fortunately, this is a rare complication.

If the catheter tip is not placed correctly, the very forceful ejection of dye will tear the lining of the vessel or "dissect" the lining away from the rest of the artery, possibly damaging the vessel irreversibly.

Some patients will have a violent sensitivity reaction to the dye with a fall in blood pressure and disturbance of heart action.

In a well-organized catheterization laboratory with a qualified cardiologist performing the test the risk of coronary arteriography is about 0.1% or less. Thus as a very rough figure about one person out of every thousand undergoing the procedure may be expected to die of it. Other complications include myocardial infarction and strokes; there may also be minor complications such as bleeding around the site where the artery is punctured to introduce the catheter and injury to nerves in the area.

The total expense of left heart catheterization and coronary arteriography, including the cardiologist's fee, the laboratory charges, and an overnight stay in the hospital will usually be about $2000.

By way of contrast, the risk of treadmill testing is .01%, that is, one person in ten thousand will die of the procedure, and the average cost is $100 to $150. Thus compared with exercise tolerance testing coronary arteriography is ten times as expensive and involves ten times the risk. It gives information that cannot be obtained by exercise testing or by any other means presently available, but the cost in dollars and in hazard to the patient is substantial.

Coronary arteriography and, indeed, catheterization of the left side of the heart in general are very skilled operations which should be carried out only by a cardiologist who has had specific training in an approved teaching institution in this particular technique. A cardiologist who is going to perform coronary arteriography or any kind of left heart catheterization should have as part of his training a minimum of six months intensive work in a busy catheterization laboratory; a year is probably a more realistic figure, and some authorities would require two. Coronary arteriography and left heart catheterization should be carried out only in a laboratory where a great many tests are performed with a team of experienced, skilled nurses and technicians; these procedures should be performed only by cardiologists who perform a large number every month and every year because the complications, when they occur, can be swift and deadly and call for rapid expert judgment. In fact, unless a cardiologist performs a number of these procedures every month, he probably should not perform them at all. The patient should feel very free to ask about the qualifications and daily performance of the personnel proposing to perform catheterization of the left side of the heart. (See the discussion on pp. 76 to 78 about which conditions justify performance of coronary arteriography and which do not.)

TREATMENT OF CORONARY ARTERY DISEASE

Coronary atheromatosis per se is probably not treatable; once an atheroma has formed there is no magic medicine known at this time that will make it shrivel up and go away. There is some speculation about whether or not these masses can regress and disappear, and in a few cases it has been claimed that this has in fact happened as a result of various diets or medications. This is in the realm of research, however, and there are no solid facts yet available. For practical purposes in 1982 an atheroma once formed is there to stay.

Medical treatment of coronary disease is based on first reducing the oxygen needs of the heart muscle to match the reduced blood supply and second on management of the various complications as they arise.

Medication
Agents that lower myocardial oxygen needs

Nitrates. In the siege of Paris in 1875 an astute physician noticed that workers hauling cases of dynamite to the barricades complained of headaches and flushing in the face, together sometimes with a sensation of pounding of the heart. The reaction he observed is called the "nitritoid" reaction, and it is the mainstay of medical treatment of angina pectoris. A tiny amount of nitroglycerin (about $\frac{1}{150}$th of a grain, or 4 milligrams) is absorbed directly into the circulation by placing it in the mouth. (If swallowed, nitroglycerin does no good.) When the patient with anginal pain takes a tablet of nitroglycerin, a distinct flushing of the face and pounding in the head will be noted, usually with the disappearance of the pain. The reason nitroglycerin works is that the medication dilates the veins all over the body; instead of returning to the heart to be pumped, a great deal of blood is held back in this reservoir of veins, and the workload on the heart drops abruptly. The bloodflow through the narrowed artery has a chance to catch up with the demand and the acute problem is over. It was thought previously that nitroglycerin worked by dilating the coronary arteries, but this happens only if the medication is injected directly into the vessel through a catheter. The principal action of nitroglycerin and other nitrates is on the veins.

Nitroglycerin relieves pain; it can also prevent it. Taken before exercise, nitroglycerin prevents the appearance of pain by lowering the workload on the heart during the exertion, thus preventing the small circulatory crisis in the heart muscle. The patient with angina pectoris who is using nitroglycerin or other quick-acting nitrates should learn to use the medicine as much as possible for *prevention* of anginal crises rather than for treating the disorder after it has occurred.

The action of nitroglycerin is very short; it wears off in ten or fifteen minutes, although one or two tablets will usually be enough for any particular anginal episode. Longer acting nitrates are available and in recent years have come into wide use.

Isosorbide, if taken under the tongue or chewed, produces an effect at least four or five times as long as nitroglycerin. It is now known that isosorbide taken in rather large amounts orally (swallowed) will exert a favorable effect on the circulation like nitroglycerin. However, because the substance is swallowed and absorbed into the bloodstream at a relatively steady rate, this effect will be prolonged for many hours, possibly all through the day and night. Large doses of isosorbide taken by mouth every six hours are an important part of treatment of many anginal syndromes.

Beta blockers. The beta-blocking drugs have opened whole new possibilities in the medical management of coronary artery disease. They may be a major reason for the fall in the coronary death rate in the last few years. These drugs work by blocking some of the effects of the sympathetic nerve endings in the tissues of the heart. The whole subject is very technical, but the end result of this kind of blocking is the production of a slower, more efficient heart. With beta blockade the heart muscle needs less oxygen to perform any given amount of work, and hence the anginal patient can safely do more work before pain or other symptoms are noticed. It is often possible to double the amount of activity that can be permitted when the patient is taking a beta-blocking drug. This means that many patients who are severely limited in their activities by anginal pain can pursue their usual gainful employments and can follow a reasonably normal lifestyle. The most commonly used of the beta-blocking drugs is propranolol.

Like all potent medicines the beta-blocking drugs have a significant toxicity and will manifest certain undesirable side effects. They cannot, for example, be used in a patient with asthma, and if taken in excessive dosage, they will produce an unacceptably slow pulse rate, or a low blood pressure. In balance, however, the undesirable effects of these drugs are far outweighed by their enormous benefits.

Calcium-blocking drugs

Earlier in the chapter it was pointed out that spasm of coronary arteries may play a role in some types of angina. It is even possible that spasm may be important in some myocardial infarctions. A totally new class of drugs based on the blocking of movement of calcium ions in the tissue is now being applied in the treatment of coronary artery disease. The Prinzmetal type of angina was the first logical application of these drugs because spasm of the vessel rather than the formation of atheromas is often the cause of this particular syndrome. Since then the calcium-blocking drugs have been found to be useful in some cases of angina associated with actual organic disease of the vessels. These drugs are still in the experimental stage and much remains to be learned, but there is no doubt that they will play an important role in the medical management of coronary artery disease. Again, there are important toxic side effects; the calcium-blocking drugs, for example, depress left ventricular function and may drop blood pressure unacceptably. (There is rarely an unmixed blessing in the use of powerful medical agents.)

General measures: how the patient lives

One of the most important parts of the treatment of coronary artery disease is readjustment of the patient's daily activities to bring them in line with the capabilities of the heart; it is also extremely important to withdraw toxic substances from the patient's environment that may provoke attacks of angina or hasten the progress of the coronary artery disease.

Physician and patient together should discuss employment; recreational activities; habits of exercise, eating, and rest and come to an agreement on the kind of living activities that are acceptable and safe for the patient. Cigarettes should be strictly forbidden, although other forms of tobacco, that is, pipes and cigars, are probably harmless. The amount of caffeine taken daily in the form of coffee or cola drinks should be strictly regulated because caffeine elevates heart rate, thus increasing the oxygen needs of the heart muscle. The amount of alcohol consumed should be discussed; there is evidence that moderate use of alcohol may be beneficial in its effect on some of the blood fats, but there is no question that excessive drinking is harmful and can even threaten life in patients with significant coronary disease.

The question of participation in an organized exercise program should be thoroughly discussed. The level of sexual activity practically always comes up and should be frankly addressed.

The diet prescription will depend on the level of fats circulating in the patient's blood, and here again the physician and patient should have complete understanding and a comprehensive prescription for food intake. (The whole subject of diet, blood fats, cholesterol, and calories is discussed on pp. 00 to 00.)

Treatment of complications

Myocardial infarction, of course, is treated with immediate bedrest in a special unit in a hospital where the heartbeat can be monitored continuously. Detection and treatment of potentially fatal disorders of rhythm is one of the prime justifications of special coronary care units. Because ventricular fibrillation is one of the commonest and most dangerous of arrhythmias associated with myocardial infarction, a specific medication, lidocaine, will be given by vein to prevent any ventricular ectopic firing. It has been shown that ventricular ectopic firing is the trigger that leads to ventricular fibrillation, and one widely accepted school of thought emphasizes preventing any ventricular ectopic firing as far as possible after a myocardial infarct. The drug lidocaine given by vein is very effective for this purpose. It is quite safe, it is rapidly excreted from the body after it is discontinued, and in a number of studies it has been shown to completely prevent primary ventricular fibrillation following a myocardial infarct. In some coronary care units it is policy to give lidocaine routinely to all patients with myocardial infarcts, while in others the procedure is to wait until ventricular ectopic firing appears and then give the drug. Either method is acceptable. Lidocaine can be given only by vein, although preparations may be available in the near future that can be given by mouth.

The length of stay in the coronary care unit will vary, but it will probably never be less than three days and with severe infarcts may be as much as a week or more.

A myocardial infarct complicated by cardiogenic shock, congestive failure, or both will often require insertion of a special type of catheter into the pulmonary artery and needles into arteries in the arm or leg to permit direct measurement of arterial blood pressure. Pulmonary artery pressures will give the physician important information about the balance in fluid load entering and leaving the heart. Direct measurement of the general arterial blood pressure is necessary because in complicated cases of congestive heart failure and shock, conventional sphygmomanometer cuff blood pressure reading may be quite unreliable. Congestive heart failure can be treated by the usual means of digitalis compounds, diuretics which drain excess water out through the kidneys, or by chemicals that dilate the arteries thereby lowering the resistance to the ejection of blood out of the left ventricle.

Failure of conduction from atria to ventricles, that is, heart block (Chapter 14) is a complication of myocardial infarction. A temporary pacemaker can be inserted without much difficulty, and the heart can be driven electronically while the conducting tissues heal.

Intermediate coronary syndrome will require the same initial care as a myocardial infarct; indeed, at first the two cannot be distinguished. Once blood tests and electrocardiographic changes have shown that a true infarct is not present the stay in the coronary care unit and the hospital itself can be considerably shortened.

Crescendo angina is also a legitimate reason for immediate hospitalization; once the physician is sure that an infarct has not occurred, he will usually treat the patient with a combination of beta-blocking drugs, vasodilators, and other supportive measures.

Surgical treatment of coronary atheromatosis

There are two kinds of surgical treatment of coronary atheromatosis. The more complex is called coronary artery bypass grafting. The simplest involves catheterization.

Coronary angioplasty

A fine catheter is threaded into a coronary artery past the point of atheromatosis and then a tiny balloon is inserted, which distends the vessel and "opens it up." The technique works surprisingly well; you would expect this kind of forcible distention to rupture the vessel and cause damage, but the manipulation of the catheter and the distention by the balloon actually help to break up the atheroma and cause it to disappear. The technique can be used in only a few cases when there is a single atheroma quite close to the beginning of the vessel so that the catheter can reach it; but among patients in whom the technique can be applied, the success ratio is about 60% (Fig. 6-14). Because most coronary atheromatosis involves multiple lesions and multiple vessels and the lesions are often quite far down the vessel out of reach of a catheter, it is obvious that this technique can be beneficial in only a small, select group of patients.

Coronary artery bypass grafting

When the coronary atheromas are not too far from the beginning of the arteries, it is possible to put a "detour" around the narrowing in the coronary artery (Fig. 6-15). The technique is in theory quite simple; a vein is taken out of a

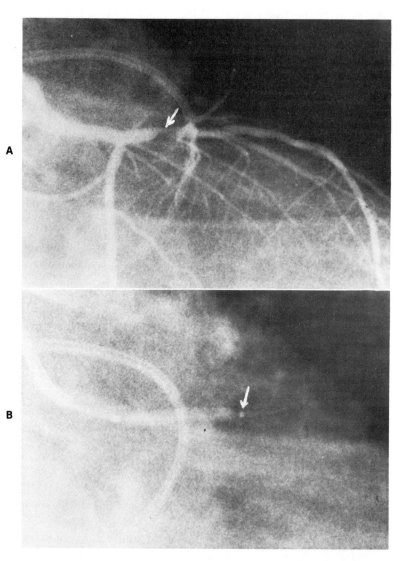

Fig. 6-14. Angioplasty. **A,** Angiogram showing severe narrowing of coronary artery *(arrow).* **B,** Angioplasty catheter threaded into and through narrowed region.

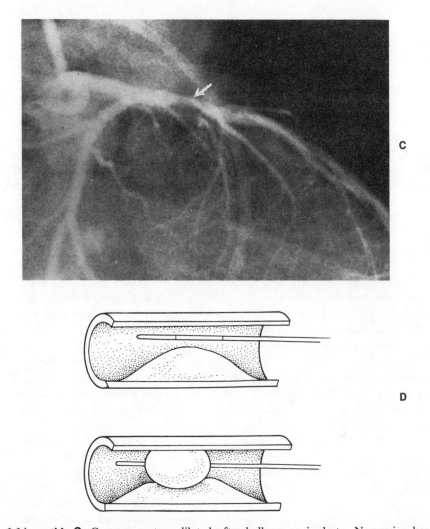

C

D

Fig. 6-14 cont'd. C, Coronary artery dilated after balloon angioplasty. Narrowing has almost disappeared. **D,** Large-scale drawing of balloon angioplasty catheter in a coronary artery. The balloon is being dilated and is compressing the atheromatous mass. (Photographs courtesy of Dr. Dietmar Gann, Tuscon, Arizona.)

Fig. 6-15. Coronary artery bypass grafting. The dotted lines indicated the vein grafts that carry blood from the aorta past the point of occlusion or blockage in the coronary arteries.

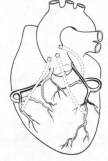

leg or sometimes out of an arm, and attacked to the aorta, where a new hole is made to receive it. This vein is then stitched into the coronary artery past the point of obstruction; thus an entirely new vessel is created that at least initially is free of obstruction and should be able to deliver a normal flow of blood to the imperiled tissue.

Multiple grafts can be inserted; as many as four or five are often placed at a single operation. The possibility of bypass grafting is limited to patients who have lesions relatively close to the origin of a coronary artery with healthy vessels beyond the point of obstruction. If a patient has many areas of obstruction all the way down the course of one or more vessels, there is no point in bypassing one lesion only to have the flow of blood obstructed by the next and the next and the next.

There is no question that in the properly selected patient coronary bypass grafting is very helpful. It often relieves anginal pain and in some cases appears to prolong life.

There are many unanswered questions about this technique, however, and questions about the usefulness and limitations of coronary bypass grafting have stirred the greatest storm of controversy in twentieth century cardiology. Anybody contemplating this kind of procedure should be thoroughly aware of the risks, complications, and benefits.

Surgical risk. Coronary bypass grafting should be carried out only by a skilled cardiac surgeon who has had very thorough training in the technique. The operation should be performed in a center where many of these procedures are carried out every week and every month. The nurses and other technical support personnel must be a well-drilled team ready to cope with any of the emergencies that frequently arise.

The death rate during or immediately after coronary bypass surgery depends, among other factors, on the efficiency of the pumping action of the heart before surgery and the location of the coronary atheromas. With a well-functioning left ventricle coronary artery bypass surgery can be carried out with a risk of about 2.5%, although in some centers it may range somewhat higher. With poor ventricular function prior to surgery the mortality will be much higher, rarely less than 10%. Surgery on the left-main artery is more dangerous with reported mortalities ranging from 10% to 30% in various institutions.

Complications

1. Myocardial infarction during or immediately after surgery. Myocardial infarction takes place in about 15% of all cases reported from practically every institution performing a large number of bypass procedures. There is some evidence to suggest that the myocardial infarction suffered during surgery is not as dangerous as one that takes place spontaneously, but there is no question that these infarcts do cause the loss of a significant amount of myocardium.

2. "Plugging" of the grafts. When the vein grafts are first placed, there is almost always a satisfying rush of blood through them; unfortunately, in a significant number of patients this does not last very long. From 20% to 30% of vein grafts will be stopped up, or occluded, about six months after bypass surgery. The veins may be occluded by a blood clot, or the cells lining the veins may simply

thicken and grown in concentric rings until they stop up the vessel completely. After the first year, about 2.8% of all grafts implanted will close each year.

3. Acceleration of disease in bypassed vessels. A curious effect of bypassing a coronary artery is that in the original vessel, "upstream" from the site of the graft, atheromatosis is enormously accelerated. About seven out of nine bypassed vessels in some studies were found to have closed off completely six months after bypass surgery. If the graft remains open, of course, this hardening of the original vessel is not particularly important, but if the graft closes, the patient's condition will have been a great deal worse.

Benefits of surgery

1. Relief of pain. In various studies it has been reported that at least three-quarters of patients operated on for relief of angina actually were relieved of their symptoms in whole or in great part as a result of bypass surgery. There is therefore little argument that a patient with angina pectoris that cannot be controlled by medical means is a logical candidate for bypass grafting if conditions in the heart are appropriate.

2. Survival. Do patients live any longer as a result of coronary bypass surgery? To answer this question the patient must first understand the risk of the disease without surgery as a basis for comparison.

One way of describing the risk of coronary artery disease is to correlate the annual death rate with the amount of abnormality in the coronary arteries.

A number of studies have reached substantially the same conclusion—in the untreated patient the natural course of coronary disease can be summarized like this:

a. Disease of the left-main coronary artery (greater than 50% narrowing of the vessel); *risk is 11% per year, cumulative.* This means that of every hundred people with significant left-main coronary artery lesions, eleven will be dead at the end of one year, twenty-two at the end of the second year, and so on. Thus in five years over 55% of patients with significant left-main coronary artery disease will die unless some intervention changes their outlook.

b. Disease of all three coronary arteries, that is, the left circumflex, the left anterior descending, and the right, approximately the same annual mortality—about 11% per year.

c. Disease of any two of the three coronary arteries; risk is about 7% per year.

d. Disease of either of the left coronary arteries, that is, the left anterior descending artery or the left circumflex artery; risk is approximately 4% per year.

e. Disease of the right coronary artery alone; risk is 2.8% per year.

You don't have to be much of a mathematician to realize that isolated disease of the right coronary artery does not pose an overwhelming risk. A 2.8% annual mortality is what most of the population over 50 has to expect in any case from all causes. Single-vessel disease involving either of the two left coronary arteries again is not particularly ominous. With disease of any two vessels about 70% of patients will be alive in five years and 30% to 35% will have died. With disease of the left-main coronary artery or of all three vessels the mortality becomes really significant, and it is in this group that coronary artery surgery might be expected to prolong life.

In estimating the risk of coronary artery disease the cardiologist must consider other factors besides the number of vessels involved. Poor left ventricular function manifested as decreased exercise tolerance or clinically evident congestive heart failure greatly increases the risk of any given coronary artery lesion. Conduction defects in the ventricular activating system, previous myocardial infarction, and increased age all diminish chances of survival. The thoughtful clinician will always balance every measurable index of risk before deciding for or against coronary bypass surgery.

It has been extraordinarily difficult to get valid research data to answer the vital question of survival with coronary bypass surgery because many other factors enter into the equation, such as poor left ventricular function or block of the conducting system within the ventricles. It has also been difficult to compare medically treated groups with surgically treated groups simply because the patients with poor left ventricular function and other complications are often relegated to medical care, while the patients selected for surgery are those who present a better risk.

Analyzing a great mass of contradictory data, most cardiologists familiar with the subject will agree with several statements about prolongation of life with coronary artery bypass surgery. First, there is no question that surgery on patients with left-main coronary artery disease prolongs life; this is particularly true if the patient has associated disease of the right coronary artery. Second, there are some studies that suggest that life is prolonged by coronary bypass surgery in the group with three-vessel disease; there is not complete unanimity of opinion on this point. Third, there are no data to show that life is prolonged by coronary artery bypass surgery with single- or double-vessel disease. (Exception: When there is a very severe lesion at the origin of the left anterior descending vessel "upstream" from the first branch leaving the artery and when treadmill tests and other studies show that this muscle is supplying a large area of heart muscle, some cardiologists think that bypass surgery may prolong life, but the data are not yet clear-cut. So far comparative studies on bypassing the left anterior descending artery have not shown any difference in survival with and without surgery.)

Who should undergo coronary artery bypass grafting? Summing up all these observations and trying to make an organized set of recommendations from them, many authorities would give the following list of reasonable indications for coronary bypass surgery:

1. Severe disabling angina pectoris that cannot be controlled by intensive medical management associated with significant disease of at least one artery. Note the words "severely disabling" and "intensive." A patient who has angina a few times a month at periods of intense physical activity but who is otherwise able to live and work normally would not be considered to have disabling angina. Similarly, intensive medical management should imply correction of all possible risk factors, management of life-style, use of vasodilators and beta-blocking drugs in adequate doses, and careful supervision by the cardiologist to be sure the

patient is really carrying out the prescribed measures. Only when these measures fail and when the angina is severe enough to curtail the patient's living activities significantly should surgery be considered.

2. Significant narrowing of the left-main coronary artery.

3. Disease of all three major coronary arteries associated with some manifestation of clinical coronary disease (angina, myocardial infarct, or intermediate coronary syndrome) and only moderate impairment of left ventricular function. The reason for the qualifications is that severe impairment of ventricular function in the presence of three-vessel disease makes the risk of surgery unacceptable, while the mere presence of three-vessel disease without symptoms and without any impairment of ventricular function does not constitute an indication for surgery.

These are the recommendations of the Council on Scientific Affairs of the American Medical Association as reported in 1979; they are still valid criteria for the justification of coronary artery bypass surgery.

Who should not have coronary artery bypass grafts?

1. Asymptomatic patients without involvement in the left-main coronary artery. A typical example of this kind of improper surgery occurs when an asymptomatic patient in vigorous good health goes to see a cardiologist for a "heart check" and as a result of treadmill testing and coronary arteriography is found to have two- or three-vessel disease. There are no data to support bypass grafting in this group of patients. Surgery in patients like this would have to be considered research and should be carried out only as part of investigative protocol in a center equipped to do experimental work.

2. Patients with single-vessel disease with no symptoms or symptoms easily controlled with medical management.

3. Patients with acute myocardial infarction or in the acute stage of unstable angina. There is no evidence to support "emergency" coronary bypass grafting in either of these categories of disease. In fact, a national cooperative study of unstable angina showed that conservative medical management produced exactly the same results as surgical management at the end of one year. Bypass grafting during the acute stage of a myocardial infarction must be considered an experimental procedure; at this time there are no data to show that it is of any benefit.

4. Patients with severe congestive heart failure as a manifestation of coronary artery disease. There are no consistent data to show that coronary bypass grafts improve ventricular function. There have been a great many contradictory studies of this subject, and the whole topic of possible improvement of function by coronary bypass grafting is still in the realm of research.

5. Patients with Prinzmetal angina caused by arterial spasm. These patients have usually done very poorly with coronary artery bypass grafting because the tendency to spasm persists in other areas of the arteries and the normal flow through the patient's own vessels leads to a high rate of closure of the grafts within a short time.

6. Patients in whom age or other diseases makes the risk of coronary bypass surgery unacceptably high.

Who should undergo cardiac arteriography?

This section comes after the discussion of coronary artery surgery for a good reason—the principal value of coronary arteriography is the selection of those patients with coronary artery disease who might benefit from coronary artery bypass grafting. There will always be a large number of patients with known coronary artery disease who should not be considered for coronary bypass surgery (1) because they are too old to undergo this procedure safely, or (2) because they have other disease that makes surgery too hazardous (severe disease of the lungs or kidneys, for example), or (3) because their symptoms are mild and easily controlled by medical management. There is no justification for performance of coronary arteriography in this group of patients, that is, patients with known coronary artery disease who are not candidates for bypass surgery. No matter what the findings are the treatment would still be the same—medical management of symptoms and control of "risk" factors.

Sometimes it is reasonable to perform coronary arteriography when a patient has pain that suggests coronary artery disease even though all the usual tests are negative. In cases like this the patient should be sure that a very thorough study has been carried out by all other means before the decision for coronary arteriography is made. The classic example of this kind of situation would be the airline pilot who suffered from suspicious chest pain but had a normal electrocardiogram and normal treadmill exercise test. The nature of the pilot's occupation would make it vital to know whether coronary disease was or was not present; coronary arteriography would be justified.

There may be "mental" or "socioeconomic" reasons for performance of coronary arteriography as well. I have seen patients with normal hearts who were so convinced that they had coronary artery disease that they made themselves invalids and made life miserable for everyone around them; only the demonstration of normal coronary arteries by angiogram cured the cardiac neurosis. Sometimes, too, coronary arteriography is needed to clear up a mistaken diagnosis of coronary artery disease by a previous physician; this kind of wrong diagnosis can change a patient's employment, destroy insurability, and cast a pall over an entire life. The demonstration of normal coronary arteries may be worth the risk and expense of arteriography in these cases.

Since practically every patient with coronary artery disease will have to confront the question of coronary arteriography, the criteria for justification for this procedure deserve detailed discussion. Here in Tucson a committee of cardiologists drew up a list of reasonable indications for the procedure at the request of a federal review agency. They also listed a number of clinical conditions and findings that did not justify the procedure. I had the privilege of serving as chairman of this committee and may be prejudiced, but I think these are fair, thoughtful statements that should be available to any patient contemplating coronary arteriography.

Indications for coronary arteriography

1. Medically intractable angina; this is further defined as angina which persists despite vigorous and adequate medical therapy. Medically intractable

angina should be differentiated from stable angina by the level of effort required to produce it and the severity of symptoms. Thus intractable angina would imply angina that appears at a level of effort that significantly limits a patient's lifestyle and normal activities. Angina that was precipitated only be very strenuous exertion far above and beyond the patient's usual and customary activity would not constitute medically intractable angina.

2. Recent history of unstable angina. This is not universally agreed on, but there is a body of competent opinion that holds that it is worth studying all patients after an episode of unstable angina because many of them appear to require coronary bypass surgery in a year or less for subsequent intractable angina. An equally qualified group insists that the proper course is to wait and see what the patient's clinical course will be and intervene only if intractable angina actually appears. There is no difference in survival with or without bypass surgery in patients following unstable angina.

3. Exercise treadmill test with 2 millimeters or greater ST depression, fall in blood pressure during exercise, severe angina and ischemic ST change at low level of exertion, or any combination of these findings. (Patients with this kind of response to treadmill testing have an increased risk of left-main or three-vessel coronary disease; they will also predictably not do well with medical management, hence investigation for possible surgery is reasonable.)

4. Myocardial infarction, typical angina pectoris, or other characteristic manifestation of coronary artery disease in a young person (arbitrarily defined as under 50—some would say under 40). Study in these cases is sometimes considered justified because a relatively young individual confronted with coronary artery disease has many decisions to make about employment, family commitments, and the possibility of improved survival with coronary bypass surgery; coronary arteriography may be essential to all these decisions.

5. Chest discomfort consistent with angina or suggestive of angina in a patient in whom careful clinical and noninvasive studies have been negative. Thorough study should be documented before arteriography would be justified and the pain should be severe enough to constitute a genuine threat to the patient's normal function; alternatively, the patient's employment may demand clarification of the diagnosis (the airline pilot again).

6. With return of symptoms after coronary bypass surgery to see if the grafts have become stopped up.

7. Need to establish coronary artery condition in a patient being evaluated for heart surgery for some other abnormality.

Clinical findings and criteria that do not justify coronary arteriography are as follows:

1. Patients with no symptoms or clinical manifestations of coronary artery disease who manifest minimal change during treadmill exercise testing. (An example would be a patient without symptoms, with good exercise tolerance, who shows 0.5 to 1 millimeter ST depression in the electrocardiogram during treadmill testing.)

2. Patients with nonspecific electrocardiographic abnormalities without any clinical manifestation of coronary artery disease.

3. Patients with chest discomfort that is by its character clearly not anginal, without any objective abnormality to suggest coronary artery disease.

4. Patients over 50 years of age surviving myocardial infarction with good functional state and with no angina or other manifestation of ischemic heart disease.

5. Stable angina pectoris that does not limit living activities significantly with good functional state in cardiac terms.

6. Patients in whom age or sex makes presence of coronary disease extremely unlikely (females before the menopause, males under 35).

7. Patients in whom age or other disease makes risk of coronary bypass surgery unacceptably high and coronary arteriography therefore irrelevant.

"Improved survival": what does it mean in years?

Earlier in the chapter it was pointed out that some patients with left-main coronary disease or three-vessel disease may live longer as the result of coronary bypass surgery. How *much* longer? Since coronary bypass surgery has been performed only for the past few years—not more than ten—it's impossible to give a really long-range answer to this question, but some figures are available. The best controlled studies comparing treated groups of patients with these two types of lesions suggest that at the end of five years, patients with left-main or three-vessel disease, especially if they have poor ventricular function, face a risk of over 50% mortality. Coronary bypass surgery appears to lower this risk to the range of about 20%. In other words, of 100 patients with severe left-main or three-vessel disease and moderate impairment of ventricular function, about fifty-five would die within five years. If these patients underwent coronary bypass surgery, only twenty of them would die. Improved survival with single- or double-vessel disease has not yet been demonstrated.

PREVENTION OF CORONARY ARTERY DISEASE

So far this chapter has described the diagnosis and treatment of established coronary artery disease. The technology of coronary arteriography, exercise stress testing, and coronary bypass surgery is dazzling, but the patient is to remember that it's all only a means of palliation—that is, lessening the effects of established disease by controlling symptoms, making possible greater physical activity, and in some cases prolonging life or at least reducing the risk of sudden death by a factor of 30% over a five-year period.

In real human worth prevention of the disease process in the first place is a thousand times more important than any other consideration. The patient may wonder why billions of dollars are spent on patching up the end stage of a disease, whereas comparatively small amounts of money and effort are devoted to preventing it in the first place. The grim medicosocioeconomic fact is that in our culture nobody is paid very much for preventing disease, whereas physicians make millions for controlling symptoms or prolonging life for a few years. The physician who works at prevention does so out of a moral sense of some basic dedication to mankind, certainly not out of any hope of gain.

Can coronary atheromatosis be prevented?

Nobody really knows the basic cause for the formation of atheromas in the coronary arteries; by the same token, nobody really knows how to prevent their formation, at least not totally.

There is a cheerier side to this depressing coin, however; certain habits and conditions of life have been identified that without any question increase the *risk* of coronary artery disease significantly. These "risk factors" have been thoroughly documented; some of them can be minimized, and some can be removed from the environment entirely.

Risk factors for coronary artery disease (Fig. 6-16)

Cigarette smoking. Everything else being equal, smoking a package or more of cigarettes a day increases the risk of death from coronary artery disease about 300%. Some statisticians give the increased risk a value of 250%, or 2.5 times, but the 300% figure is probably reasonable. Therefore the person who smokes a package of cigarettes a day is three times as likely to die of coronary disease as the one who does not when all other risk factors have been equalized. *This is unnecessary risk and totally correctable!*

Heredity. There is no question that the tendency toward formation of atheromas in the coronary arteries is genetically transmitted. If both parents have coronary artery disease before age 70, the risk for their children goes up 1.5 to 2 times. To put it another way, the risk increases about 200%.

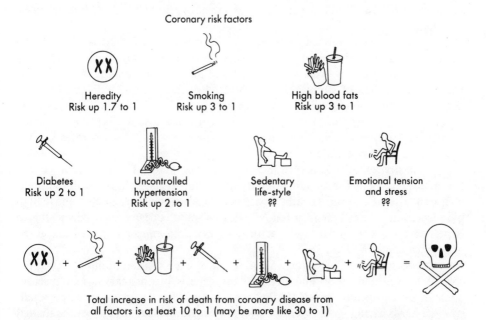

Total increase in risk of death from coronary disease from all factors is at least 10 to 1 (may be more like 30 to 1)

Fig. 6-16. Total increase in risk of death from coronary disease from all factors is at least 10 to 1 (maybe more like 30 to 1).

The variation in genetic risk is very striking in isolated ethnic groups like the Indians of Arizona. The Navajo and Papago tribes, for example, have very little coronary disease, no matter how much fat they eat or how much they smoke. (In three years of conducting cardiac clinics all over the Navajo reservation I saw one case of clinical coronary artery disease; it was in a 75-year-old medicine man who had walked 25 miles to see me.)

A young couple with heavy coronary artery heredity on both sides should certainly approach marriage and begetting children very cautiously.

Hypertension. Uncontrolled high blood pressure increases the risk of coronary disease by a factor of at least 2, or 200%. When hypertension is controlled medically, the increased risk appears to be completely eliminated, and the well-controlled hypertensive faces no greater risk than his normotensive fellow. *This is a controllable risk; it can be almost totally eradicated.*

High blood fats. Elevation of total blood fats increases the risk of coronary death by about 200%. An elevated cholesterol level is the most important risk factor, while a high triglyceride level, although increasing risk, is not as ominous as a high cholesterol level. There is apparently a different risk, depending on levels of "good" (high density) and "bad" (low density) cholesterol-protein combinations. (See pp. 88 to 92.) *This is a partially controllable risk.*

Diabetes. The presence of diabetes probably doubles the risk of coronary artery disease and coronary artery death. Very careful control of blood-sugar levels in diabetes may cut down on coronary complications, but this has not yet been proved to everybody's satisfaction. Even with careful control diabetics still face increased risk, but there is some data to show that if the blood sugar is maintained near normal levels, the risk may be substantially reduced. *This is a partially controllable risk.*

Sex. For some reason that nobody understands the female is protected by her hormones until the menopause; in other words, it is extremely rare to discover clinical coronary artery disease in a woman while she is still having menstrual periods. A great deal of study has been devoted to the possible linkage of the sex hormones with fat metabolism and other risk factors for coronary disease, but all we can say at this point is that the risk of coronary disease in premenopausal women is extremely low; after menopause the risk rapidly accelerates until it equals that of comparable men.

Obesity. Obesity is not an independent risk factor. There are many excellent medical reasons for avoiding obesity, but being overweight per se does not increase the risk of coronary death. Obese people are much more likely to have high blood pressure than their thin fellows; in this sense, obesity by predisposing to hypertension is a secondary risk factor. *This is a secondary risk factor and completely controllable.*

Emotional tension: stress. Volumes have been written about the possible role of mental and emotional stress in the genesis of coronary artery disease. Some investigators have proposed that there is a specific coronary-prone personality—the hard-driving, goal-oriented, overworking individual who is never satisfied with previous accomplishments. The data on this continue to be very conflicting, and for every study correlating mental stress or occupational tensions with increased coronary disease, there is another study that proves just the opposite.

As a general health recommendation any physician would agree that excessive fatigue and emotional stress should be minimized and that anybody is better off with periods of rest, relaxation, and recreation, but no investigator at this time can state with any certainty that emotional stress predisposes to coronary atheromatosis or its complications.

Exercise. I am personally in favor of exercise, partake of it regularly, and find most forms of strenuous exertion very pleasant. The joggers and tennis players who grunt and sweat under a heavy self-imposed load do so partly because they enjoy their exercise, but partly because there is a widespread notion that good physical conditioning and sustained exercise help prevent coronary artery disease. Unfortunately, this is not true. The massive data about exercise and coronary disease can best be summarized by this statement: there is no evidence to show that exercise in any form, taken over any period, prevents the formation of coronary atheromas. There is suggestive evidence to show that people who exercise regularly and maintain good physical condition will experience the clinical manifestations of the disease later and possibly tolerate them better. Certainly the human animal through its two million years of recent evolution has been a physically active creature adapted for the hunter-gatherer society in which running and strenuous exertion were a part of daily life. It's reasonable to assume that our endocrine glands and the assorted chemicals of our body are in tune with a life that involves strenuous physical activity for considerable periods every day and that the absence of this kind of activity is probably deleterious. Therefore as a cardiologist I advise patients to become involved in sane programs of conditioning and exercise, not with the expectation that this will prevent disease of the coronary arteries but with the hope that the disease will appear later and involve less risk when it does become manifest.

Age. The one risk factor impossible to influence is the passage of time. Coronary artery disease is extremely rare in young individuals (men under 35, women before menopause) and increases in almost linear fashion in the 50s and 60s. Coronary artery disease is by far the leading single cause of death in males over 50.

The Western World as a risk factor: environmental toxins. Something about the kind of culture and the way of life we call "Western" predisposes to coronary artery disease. In any Third World nation that adopts the dubious blessings of Western civilization the coronary death rate invariably rises. Why? What does it? Cigarettes? The pace of our lives? What we eat? Our relative sloth? Nobody really knows, but beyond any question something inherent in our civilization is killing us.

The great Paul Dudley White, the dean of American cardiology, pointed out that the rise in the use of automobiles kept pace with the rise in coronary death rates. He may have been more perceptive than anyone realized. Studies on the Los Angeles freeways have shown that the inhalation of carbon monoxide lowers the oxygen-carrying capacity of blood to the danger point in patients with coronary artery disease. When patients with documented angina pectoris sit quietly in a car being transported through polluted freeway air, their continously recorded electrocardiogram shows the same injury current that it would show if they were walking on a treadmill to the point of ischemic change. This is a prolonged effect; after an hour's ride on a polluted freeway the exercise tolerance of an anginal patient is cut in half; even as much as two hours after leaving the freeway the patient can conduct only half as much treadmill exercise without pain or electrocardiographic change as he could before he started his trip. Carbon monoxide reduces the capacity of the hemoglobin in the blood to carry oxygen; when the oxygen supplied to an area of heart muscle is already reduced because of coronary disease, this further compromise of oxygen delivery may threaten the survival of the area of heart muscle involved. For example, an executive has hardening of several coronary arteries but he doesn't know it yet; so far there have been no symptoms. He drives home through a polluted atmosphere and the carbon monoxide lowers the oxygen-carrying capacity of his blood past the danger point for some time after he leaves the freeway. He goes for a brisk swim or mows the lawn and then either falls dead or suffers a myocardial infarct. This man is in a very direct sense a victim of the polluted environment generated by the needlessly foul exhaust of thousands of internal combustion engines.

This is only one of a thousand toxic threats in our environment; in combinations and permutations many of them may be contributing to this mysterious plague. What is certain beyond question is that by leaving the life-style of hoes and axes, of bows and spears, of leisurely progress across earth and seas in tune with the rising and setting of sun, moon, stars and by frantically pursuing symbols of wealth at ever higher speeds ever more aggressively in an increasingly foul environment, we have generated a monster more real and far more deadly than any hot-throated dragon that troubled our forebears' dreams.

CORONARY ARTERY DISEASE: SOME GUIDELINES

At this point it's time to compress a great deal of information into a few simple statements about coronary artery disease.

CAVEATS

• Coronary artery disease is by far the commonest cause of cardiac illness and death in the Western World, accounting for over half of all cardiac deaths in adult males in the United States.

• Almost all coronary artery disease is caused by *atheromatosis,* that is, formations of masses of fatty material called atheromas on the linings of the coronary arteries, interfering with the flow of blood through these vessels and sometimes stopping it completely.

• Coronary artery disease will occur in several clinical forms: (1) angina pectoris: pain in the chest noted on effort (when the heart is working harder) and relieved by rest. (2) Myocardial infarct: total stoppage of an artery with death of the heart muscle supplied by that artery (the common type of "heart attack"). (3) Intermediate coronary syndrome, or coronary insufficiency: an attack somewhere between angina pectoris and myocardial infarction in severity. (4) Unstable, or crescendo, angina: angina pectoris that suddenly becomes more severe, with more frequent pain produced by less exertion; it is always an emergency requiring hospitalization.

• Coronary artery disease can often be detected by symptoms. A skilled cardiologist will rely heavily on the history given by the patient. It may also be detected by the electrocardiogram recorded at rest or during controlled exercise. Myocardial infarction will usually be diagnosed by a combination of symptoms, progressive changes in the electrocardiogram, and rises in certain chemicals in the blood called enzymes.

Rarely, it may be necessary to inject dye into the coronary arteries with a catheter to see which arteries are diseased and how severely. This technique is chiefly used to find out whether surgery on the coronary arteries may benefit the patient. Occasionally it may be helpful in the diagnosis of coronary artery disease when suspicious symptoms are present and all other means have failed.

• Medical management of coronary artery disease includes nitroglycerin and other blood vessel–dilating drugs that "unload" the heart, beta-blocking drugs that reduce the oxygen needs of the heart muscle and make the heart a more efficient pump, calcium-blocking drugs that prevent spasm of the coronary arteries, control of risk factors known to predispose to coronary artery disease, and adjustment of life-style to the heart's capabilities.

• Known risk factors for coronary artery disease include cigarette smoking, high blood pressure, diabetes, high blood fats (principally cholesterol), heredity, age, and sex (male). A combination of medical management with adjustment of risk factors and life-style is all that is needed in a majority of cases.

• Surgical treatment includes two techniques. The first is dilating the diseased artery with a balloon on a small catheter that is actually inserted into the vessel. This can be done in only the few cases in which the narrowed part of the artery is close enough to its origin so that the catheter can reach the atheroma and break it up. Results are moderately encouraging with this new technique.

The common kind of coronary artery surgery consists of bypassing the diseased artery with a bit of vein from the patient's leg. Coronary bypass surgery has been in use for over ten years and certain facts have emerged about the results. (1) Coronary artery bypass surgery can relieve pain when medical means have failed. (2) Coronary artery surgery has been shown to prolong life only in a small percentage of patients, that is, those with disease of the left-main coronary artery or those with disease of all three coronary arteries associated with moderate impairment of function of the left ventricle as a result of their disease.

"Prolongation of life" means a 30% improvement in survival over a five-year period with the best possible results. Coronary artery disease progresses relentlessly in the other arteries that have not been bypassed unless there is strenuous medical management to arrest the process.

The chief reason for performing coronary artery bypass graft surgery, therefore, is *relief of pain that cannot be controlled by medical means.* The secondary reason is the hope of prolonging life in either of the two categories listed earlier. These two categories together constitute less than 20% of all cases of coronary artery disease. Catheterizing all patients known to have coronary artery disease to see if they fall into one of these two groups would be an enormous and unacceptable expense and risk. There are some clues to the presence of these two types of disease listed in the detailed discussion of coronary arteriography in the earlier part of this book. By following up these clues probably three quarters of all patients with surgical coronary artery disease will be discovered.

These are the bare bones facts about coronary artery disease. How do they square with what is happening in the clinical management of coronary artery disease in the United States today? Here are a few anecdotes:

A 28-year-old woman presented herself at my office last year describing chest pain that was clearly not anginal in character. She had an insignificant heart murmur of a common type associated with a common, harmless type of valve abnormality. She showed me with some pride a record of her expensive cardiac study in a Chicago hospital; the study included coronary arteriography.

It is virtually impossible for a 28-year-old female to have clinical coronary artery disease in the first place, and in the second this woman had no symptoms remotely suggestive of the disease. The study was completely unjustified.

An 82-year-old man with known angina pectoris usually controlled with medicine was advised to have heart catheterization, even though he was obviously too old for surgery, and the disease was easily controlled by simple medical management. (Fortunately this was halted in time.)

A 32-year-old man playing tennis developed pain in the muscles of his shoulder and upper chest. The pain came and went with motion of the arm and was quite clearly related to the muscles and ligaments of the shoulder girdle, a fact that could be determined with considerable accuracy by three or four questions. The young man consulted a physician who referred him to a cardiologist who recommended coronary arteriography to be carried out the next morning before any further studies had been completed. Fortunately this procedure was averted by adequate consultation.

A 70-year-old woman who had a mild myocardial infarct involving the right coronary artery (the mildest of all types of infarct) and who had an uneventful course with complete recovery and normal function without symptoms thereafter was subjected to coronary arteriography. This patient was clearly not a candidate for coronary bypass surgery because she had no symptoms at all and in fact did not even require medication to live a normal life; there was no conceivable reason why coronary arteriography should have been carried out.

A 46-year-old woman with chest pain that came and went with breathing was subjected to coronary arteriography less than eighteen hours after seeing a cardiologist, before any other studies had been done and despite the fact that the pain did not remotely suggest the pain of coronary artery disease.

These are cases from my own experience, but conversations with cardiologists throughout the country convince me they are typical; one could multiply them by 100,000 and have an accurate estimate of the true state of affairs concerning coronary arteriography in the United States today.

The annual bill for coronary arteriography, as near as it can be estimated, is probably around five hundred million dollars—for this one diagnostic procedure alone. It is the consensus of a great many competent cardiologists in the United States that 50% of the coronary arteriography procedures performed would not be justified by the standards proposed here or indeed by any reasonable standards.

It is likely that the same depressing observations apply to coronary artery bypass grafting. The annual cost of this procedure in the United States alone runs into billions of dollars. Coronary arteriography and coronary artery bypass grafting impose an enormous load on our annual health care bill. The yield is the relief of anginal pain in some cases and the prolongation of life by a few percentage points in others.

It is conservative to state that with the imposition of reasonable controls on both procedures the annual cost could be cut in half without any harmful effect on the American public.

Prevention with control of risk factors is ten times more important than surgical procedures that can only "patch up" the end stage of a disease!

The following is a suggested dialogue with your physician if he recommends coronary arteriography or coronary bypass surgery

Patient: Do you know already that I have coronary artery disease? How do you know this? If you do, why is it necessary to perform coronary arteriography?

The answer is

To see if you might benefit from coronary artery bypass graft surgery.

The dialogue might continue:

Patient: Coronary artery surgery can either relieve pain or in some cases prolong life, right? What would be the purpose in my case?

If the answer is "To relieve anginal pain," go to the next question:

Patient: Have I had a reasonable trial of medical management? Have you tried beta blockers and vasodilators? Is the anginal pain severe enough to limit my activity significantly? Does it keep me from performing acceptably in my work or in recreation?

If the answer to all these is a "yes" that both patient and physician can agree on, there is a reasonable basis to perform coronary angiography with a view to coronary bypass graft surgery. If there is no angina, the dialogue might run like this:

Patient: Is there some possibility that coronary artery surgery might prolong my life? This would only be true if I had left-vein or three-vessel disease, right? Do you have any reason to suppose I have left-vein or three-vessel disease? What reason or reasons do you have?

CAVEATS

• If the physician tells you he knows you have coronary artery disease and does not consider you a candidate for coronary bypass graft surgery but wants to perform angiography anyway—demand consultation.

• If the physician tells you he knows you have coronary artery disease and agrees that you have either mild angina or that you have not had an adequate medical trial to control anginal pain but wants to go ahead with coronary antiography and possible bypass surgery anyway, demand consultation.

• If the physician recommends surgery *on the basis of prolonging life* in the presence of single-vessel or two-vessel disease, demand consultation.

Summary of coronary bypass surgery

If coronary artery surgery is being recommended to relieve anginal pain, the patient must be very sure that the angina is severe enough to be significant and that it cannot be controlled by medical means. If the surgery is being recommended to prolong life, the patient must be very sure that he suffers from either left-vein or three-vessel disease or some reasonable equivalent thereof so that there is some prospect of improving survival by surgery.

DECLINE OF CORONARY ARTERY DISEASE

A cheerful note for the end of this chapter. For reasons that nobody quite understands the death rate from coronary artery disease has been declining in the last five years. This may be due to the greater emphasis on control of risk factors, the increasing use of unsaturated fats in our diet, the enthusiasm for exercise, and the better medical management of the disease. However, for whatever reason it appears that quite apart from the patients subjected to coronary bypass surgery the total coronary death rate, which had been rising steadily throughout the first half of the century, has shown a significant and encouraging drop every year for the past four or five years. I suggest that anybody concerned with coronary artery disease read again the section on risk factors and their management and implement as many of the recommendations as is possible; prevention is everything!

7   Diet, blood fats, cholesterol, and coronary death

"Do I have cholesterol?" "Do I have *too much* cholesterol?" "Can I eat eggs?" "What about unsaturated fats and butter?" "Do different things that I eat have anything to do with my coronary artery disease? If so, what should I eat and what shouldn't I eat?"

Every physician in the Western World has had to contend with these questions from every thoughtful, informed victim of coronary disease—indeed, from every potential victim, which includes most of the population. These are reasonable questions, and they deserve answers. They have been prompted by the flood of information, much of it conflicting, about the relationship of fat in the blood, dietary fat, and types of fat eaten to the formation of atheromas in the coronary arteries.

As initially laid down coronary atheromas are, indeed, masses of fat; they have the same percentage composition as the fats that normally circulate in the blood, strongly suggesting that the circulating blood fats are responsible for the deposits of fats on the lining of the coronary arteries.

Fats are essential to life; no one could live very long without an adequate circulating level of the appropriate fats used in the cellular metabolism. Cholesterol is a vital substance basic to the formation of the bile and to many of the hormones in the body.

The basic questions are, therefore:

1. Is an excessively high level of circulating fats of any kind a cause or a partial cause of coronary atheromatosis?
2. Specifically, is an elevated level of cholesterol in the blood related to coronary atheromatosis?
3. Does the amount of fat eaten in the diet have anything to do with the levels of fat in general and cholesterol in particular circulating in the blood?
4. Does reducing the amount of fat in the diet lower the levels of fat circulating in the blood?
5. Does lowering the levels of fat and cholesterol in the blood really prevent the formation of coronary atheromatosis or lessen the likelihood of its occurrence?

Final answers to these questions are simply not yet available. An enormous body of research is still underway which may clarify this whole set of relationships. At this time there are suggestive data and a few reasonable recommendations that can be made. To understand them, the patient must know something about the kinds of fats that circulate in the blood, the way in which they are combined, and the significance of the various types.

BLOOD FATS

The two major fats circulating in the blood are **cholesterol** and **triglycerides.** These substances are not soluble in water or blood; in their "pure" form they could not move freely through the fluids of the body or across the cell walls. To "dissolve" these fats, they are combined with protein elements into complex molecules called lipoproteins, that is, combinations of fat and proteins (the stem "lipo-" always refers to fats or fatty substances).

The significant lipoprotein fractions in terms of coronary risk are as follows:

1. Very low-density lipoproteins (VLDL). The very low-density lipoprotein molecule consists mostly of triglyceride; it is chiefly manufactured in the body and is not derived from dietary sources.

2. Intermediate-density lipoproteins (IDL). This molecule includes about equal parts of cholesterol and triglyceride.

3. Low-density lipoproteins (LDL). This molecule contains 50% cholesterol; elevation of LDL will almost always be associated with a high blood level of cholesterol. This is the specific lipoprotein molecule that has been associated with coronary artery disease statistically; in other words, individuals with an elevated LDL level have an increased risk of coronary artery disease and coronary death.

4. High-density lipoproteins (HDL). This is the "good" cholesterol that everybody has been reading about recently. Most of the publications on the subject of HDL have been accurate. In fact, there has been evidence for some years that high levels of HDL actually act as a protective mechanism against the development of coronary disease. Patients with an elevated HDL will have a high serum cholesterol, but this will not have the significance of a high serum cholesterol associated with LDL. It is especially pleasant for most people to discover that elevated HDL has been correlated with moderate ingestion of alcohol and consistent exercise. Thus several sets of tennis and a gin and tonic in the clubhouse afterward can genuinely be viewed as therapeutic!

SERUM CHOLESTEROL

Many of the early studies of the relationship of serum cholesterol to coronary artery disease were confusing because the distinction between LDL and HDL forms of lipoprotein had not been made and was not included in the studies.

What evidence exists to prove that an elevated serum cholesterol increases the risk of coronary death?

In animals, high-cholesterol diets has been consistently shown to produce a rise in serum cholesterol and an increase in the formation of atheroma in the coronaries. In species such as rabbits this can be done almost at will. Some animal species, however, resist the effect of high-cholesterol feedings and absolutely refuse either to elevate the blood cholesterol or to form atheromas. There is a difference in the way different animals—and for that matter, different humans—handle an increased cholesterol load, and this difference is clinically very important.

Population studies around the world have suggested that a high-fat, high-cholesterol intake is associated with a high level of coronary artery disease and coronary death. Conversely, groups which characteristically eat a low-fat, low-cholesterol diet appear to have a much lower risk of coronary artery disease in general. There are some important exceptions in these studies: the Masai of East Africa, for example, are a nomadic tribe who eat an extremely high-fat, high-cholesterol diet consisting chiefly of cows' blood, cows' milk, and red meat. The total cholesterol intake of these tribesmen is fantastic by any standards, and yet the level of cholesterol in their blood is low and their coronary artery death rate is one of the lowest ever studied. The Navajo and Papago tribes of Arizona have average serum cholesterols, eat a very mixed diet quite high in fat, and yet have a coronary death rate about one quarter that of the Anglo population or less. The Bantu, or black population of South Africa, were found to eat a very low-fat diet and to have low serum cholesterol levels; they also had an extremely low rate of coronary artery disease and coronary death. On reexamination, however, it was found that these tribesmen do, in fact, have atheroma formation, but it is chiefly in the aorta just where it leaves the heart rather than in the coronary arteries.

Clearly, there are enormous inborn differences in the way different individuals and different groups "handle," or metabolize, cholesterol and other fats, and these must be taken into account before deciding just what the relationship of dietary fat and dietary cholesterol is to risk of coronary death.

When a cultural group is studied with different serum cholesterol levels in individuals, it has been difficult to relate these levels to differences in intake of dietary fat. Studies in Framingham, Massachusetts, and Tecumseh County, Georgia, so far have not made any clear relationship between dietary fat intake, cholesterol intake, and serum cholesterol levels in members of any particular social or regional group. It should be emphasized, however, that these studies are incomplete and that longer term follow-up with more precise definition of dietary intake of fats may show a more clear-cut relationship.

What are the different ways that humans respond to an increased intake of cholesterol?

There are two mechanisms of response to cholesterol intake. (1) Cholesterol is normally manufactured in the liver. Even if a person ate no cholesterol at all, the liver would still continue to turn out satisfactory quantities. If an excess load of cholesterol is taken in the food, some individuals "turn off" the production of cholesterol in their livers. This is the most efficient mechanism for keeping the blood cholesterol from rising, and the individual whose body responds in this way is probably fortunate. (2) Cholesterol is excreted in the bile and in the stool. Most people, at least in the Western World, respond to an increased cholesterol load by this increased excretion mechanism, which is, unfortunately, not very efficient.

Experiments have shown that when large amounts of cholesterol are fed to individuals who can "turn off" liver production, their serum cholesterol will not rise significantly. On the other hand, when excess loads of cholesterol are fed to individuals whose bodies respond only by excretion, the serum cholesterol level may rise very dramatically.

As one distinguished student of the field has commented, "Some men behave like rabbits and monkeys, with rather massive rises in serum cholesterol in response to cholesterol feeding because of the inability to turn off liver synthesis; others behave like rats and dogs, with no rise in serum level to cholesterol feeding because of their body's ability to stop synthesis of cholesterol in the liver and increase the amount excreted in the stool."

Since people vary this much in the way their body handles an increased level or fat load, it is clear that general population studies including both types of responders can be very confusing.

What is the role of unsaturated fats?

The chemical molecule of fat consists of a long chain of carbon atoms combined with hydrogen and certain organic submolecules (fatty acids) that determine the character of the fat. If all the electric linkages on the carbon atoms are taken up by hydrogen molecules, the fat is called "saturated." Some fats, on the other hand, have electric charges on their carbon atoms which are not taken up by hydrogen, and these are, roughly speaking, referred to as "unsaturated" fats.

The intake of saturated fatty acids with between twelve and eighteen carbon atoms raise cholesterol levels very clearly in every group studied to date. Thus the ingestion of saturated fats of a particular type will quite clearly raise LDL and serum cholesterol, both significant risk factors for coronary death.

Eating large amounts of polyunsaturated fats will lower cholesterol and LDL levels, but on an equal-weight basis polyunsaturated fats will lower LDL/cholesterol levels only half as much as eating saturated fats raises them. In other words, the way to control the levels of low-density lipoprotein and its contained cholesterol is to *stop eating saturated fats;* this is much more efficient than eating large amounts of unsaturated fats. Nobody knows why eating saturated fats produces a rise in the serum cholesterol level, but the fact is established beyond any question.

What level of cholesterol is dangerous?

There is no fixed level of serum cholesterol that can be considered completely safe or necessarily lethal. The risk varies on a curve. In other words, somebody with a serum level of 350 milligrams per 100 milliliter of blood certainly has a significant risk factor for coronary artery disease and coronary death; so does the patient with a level of 215, although it is less, and so on down the curve. Levels under 200 are considered "normal" in American society, but, in fact, they may be too high in comparison with the extremely low levels found in a number of ethnic groups in the world where fat intake is very low. Possibly a serum level of 120 should be considered "normal," but, again, nobody really knows what the cutoff point is.

Has anybody really shown that cutting down fat intake and lowering serum cholesterol prevents coronary artery disease when genetic and other factors are equalized? Now yet; there are some suggestive observations, however, such as the statistics on the Seventh Day Adventists in California. Within this group there were found to be nonvegetarians, lacto-ovovegetarians (people who use milk and eggs but otherwise stick to a vegetarian diet), and complete vegetarians. The coronary heart disease mortality for these three groups compared with the general population was 34% lower, 57% lower, and 77% lower, respectively. Studies like this are strongly suggestive, of course, but they cannot be accepted as definitive scientific data yet.

WHAT SHOULD THE PATIENT WITH CORONARY DISEASE DO ABOUT DIETARY FATS; WHAT BLOOD STUDIES SHOULD BE CARRIED OUT?

Every patient with coronary artery disease deserves a careful study of the blood fats. If an abnormally high level of cholesterol or LDL is found, the physician should be very careful to be sure that there are not other diseases causing these elevated serum fat levels such as diabetes or thyroid disease. Not every laboratory is equipped to carry out these observations accurately, and the coronary patient would do well to ask some searching questions about the kind of laboratory equipment available and the level of quality control. Blood fat determinations should be carried out only when the fat intake has been stabilized for several days because a temporary high load of dietary fat can distort the results. If a patient with coronary disease is found to have a high serum cholesterol and a high LDL, then some reasonable recommendations can be made.

1. A diet relatively low in cholesterol should be prescribed (Appendix 1).
2. The percentage of saturated fats taken in the diet should be cut down as far as possible.
3. Rechecks of LDL and cholesterol levels should be carried out at reasonable intervals to see if the patient is responding to the regimen.
4. If elevated blood fat levels persist, a complete vegetarian diet may be tried. With the use of modern synthetic foods this is much more practical than it was a few years ago.
5. In extreme cases of high blood fats, particularly high blood cholesterol/ LDL levels, certain powerful drugs may be prescribed. A number of preparations have appeared on the market in recent years, all professed to lower blood fat and cholesterol, and a few of them have proved useful. Some of these drugs have had very severe toxicity and have been removed from the market, while others are marginal in their performance. Drug therapy is reserved for the difficult case with persistent high cholesterol/LDL levels and requires careful continuing medical supervision.

•   •   •

In brief summary, there is evidence around the globe to suggest that population groups that habitually eat a low-fat diet and have a low serum cholesterol level have a lower risk of coronary disease in general, although there are some striking exceptions to this rule. Some individuals have an inborn mechanism for disposing of excess cholesterol that makes them immune to the effects of a high-fat, high-cholesterol diet. These fortunate individuals simply stop producing cholesterol in their livers when too much is taken in through the diet. Most people, at least in the population groups that comprise the Western World, do not have this efficient mechanism for disposing of cholesterol and hence are more vulnerable to the effects of increased intake of cholesterol in the diet.

An elevated serum cholesterol may be found in one of two complex molecules—the low-density lipoprotein, a dangerous element clearly associated with increased risk of coronary artery disease, or the high-density lipoprotein, a benevolent substance that seems to protect against coronary artery disease. The coronary patient with an elevated serum cholesterol level should know which of these lipoproteins is actually responsible for the high cholesterol level and should discuss with the cardiologist the factors that can influence each.

It has not been clearly demonstrated that lowering serum cholesterol and LDL levels by dietary means will benefit the patient with coronary artery disease or will, in fact, prevent its appearance, but there are data to suggest that this may be the case. Lowering serum cholesterol/LDL levels by a diet low in cholesterol and saturated fats is probably harmless and may be very helpful; it seems to be a reasonable course at this time for any patient suffering from coronary artery disease who has elevated levels of these blood fats.

A NATIONAL TREND

The death rate due to cardiovascular disease of all kinds has dropped 21% in the United States between 1968 and 1976. This drop includes a significant drop in the number of deaths caused by coronary artery disease. Many factors have changed in our national environment in that time, but one of the most significant may be the lowered intake of saturated fats and the increased use of polyunsaturated vegetable oils. This change in dietary habits has been reflected by a significant fall in the average level of cholesterol in the United States population in the last ten years—about 5% to 10%. Figures like these do not constitute scientific proof, but every investigator in the field agrees that they are at least strongly suggestive that the change in our national dietary habits is resulting in fewer coronary deaths.

8   Hypertensive heart disease

The word "hypertension" means high blood pressure. (It has nothing to do with being nervous or agitated, as people often think.) A certain pressure is present in the blood vessels of the body at all times. The pressure in the arteries, naturally, is not the same every second. When the left ventricle is discharging its blood into the arteries, the pressure rises. Between beats, while the left ventricle is refilling, the pressure drops. The rise and fall of pressure in the blood vessels with each beat of the heart makes it possible to feel a pulse in the arteries of the wrist or in other parts of the body. When recording a patient's blood pressure, one measures the top pressure, that is, the pressure when the pulse wave is at the top of its curve, as in Fig. 8-1. This is the highest pressure existing within the blood vessels when the left ventricle is ejecting the peak volume of blood into the arteries. The bottom pressure of the pulse curve is also measured. This is the pressure in the arteries when the aortic valve has closed and the left ventricle is refilling. At this point no blood is being pumped out of the heart into the arteries; hence the pressure is relatively low. When the pressure is 120/80, the top pressure when the left ventricle is pumping blood into the arteries is 120 and the bottom pressure between beats when no blood is being pumped is 80.

The alert patient will ask at once, "120 what?" All pressure is measured in some kind of a unit made up to fit the measurement in question—feet, pounds, etc. The pressure in the arteries is measured by the height in millimeters of a column of mercury in a glass tube that the arterial pressure will balance or support. (A millimeter is a metric unit of measurement equal to about $\frac{1}{16}$ of an inch.) Various means are used to measure the pressure in the arteries. One could, of course, insert a hollow needle into an artery and let the blood flow into a tube connected to a pressure-measuring device. This is sometimes done, but it is not usually necessary. Ordinarily a cuff is placed around the arm and is inflated with air until the artery is compressed and shut off. Then the air is let out of this cuff until there is just enough pressure squeezing on the artery so that blood can force its way through at the peak, or top, pressure. This is called the systolic pressure because it represents the highest pressure created in the arteries by the force of left ventricular contraction. By letting more air out of the cuff, the physician can find the lowest point at which any compression at all is exerted on the artery. This is the diastolic pressure. When the physician tells a patient that his blood pressure equals one number over another, such as 130/70 or 140/90, he is simply describing the peak and valley of the pulse curve, or pressure curve, inside the arteries.

Normal blood pressure varies as much as normal height. It would be ridiculous to tell people that they should all be exactly 5 feet 11½ inches tall. It would be equally ridiculous to tell everybody they must have exactly 120 millimeters systolic pressure or 80 millimeters diastolic pressure in the arteries. One can only state what normal readings are and what the range of normal is. For most adults the systolic pressure will lie somewhere between 100 and 140 millimeters of mer-

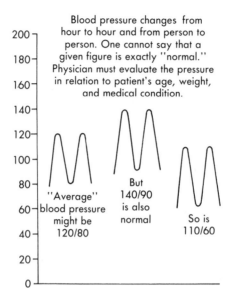

Fig. 8-1. Range of normal blood pressures.

cury. Diastolic pressure will lie between 60 and 90. An "average" reading might be 118/72, or 132/84. In young females and thin individuals it is quite common to see a systolic pressure below 100, with a correspondingly low diastolic pressure. A reading of 90/60 is common in such people. In middle-aged or older individuals it is equally common to see a systolic pressure of 140 or 150 and a diastolic pressure in the low or middle 90s. A pressure of 150/94 would not be surprising in a 60-year-old individual and would certainly not, of itself, indicate any disease.

KINDS OF HIGH BLOOD PRESSURE

High blood pressure is a symptom, like fever. It is not actually a single disease. Elevation of blood pressure may happen for many reasons. Fright or anger in normal people often causes a rise in both systolic and diastolic pressures. At complete rest the pressure tends to drop. By simply breathing deeply for a minute or two or by relaxing, an individual can cause the pressure to drop twenty or thirty points. A person's pressure will change ten, twenty, or thirty points every hour during the day, depending on whether he is running up a hill, lying on a sofa watching a television set, kissing his mate, or arguing with the boss.

Benign arteriosclerotic hypertension

The most common cause of true elevation of blood pressure, or high blood pressure, will be described first. This is simply hardening of the arteries, or as physicians put it, generalized arteriosclerosis.

Normally the arteries are quite elastic. They are something like rubber tubes, with a certain amount of "give." The elasticity of the arteries lies somewhere between that of an inner tube and a tire casing; the very larger arteries tend to be almost rigid, while the small ones are quite flexible. However, in the normal individual all arteries have a certain amount of elasticity. As the blood is pumped into the arteries from the left ventricle, the vessels distend somewhat, taking up the first shock of the outpouring blood. Between beats, when the pressure is falling, the arterial tubes constrict, or narrow. This elastic quality of the arteries tends to reduce both the upward and downward swing of the pressure curve.

In the common type of widespread hardening of the arteries seen in many individuals over 50 years of age the arteries lose some of this elastic quality. As a rule, this is a generalized "all over" kind of process, although some parts of the body such as the brain may be affected more than others. The walls of the great vessels such as the aorta become almost as hard as a garden hose, and the medium-sized arteries are almost as rigid. Systolic pressure will now be higher because the arteries cannot expand with the ejection of the blood. To understand this, the reader may picture the difference between two boxers being hit on the jaw. Imagine one boxer "rolling with the punch," falling back swiftly so that he dissipates the force of the blow. Imagine the second boxer standing flat-footed, rigid, unyielding, allowing himself to be hit as hard as possible. The difference in the effect on the two boxers is easy to imagine. The same thing is true of the force, or pressure, against the walls of the arteries when the arteries cannot yield with the outgushing blood. Instead of being 140 at its peak, the pressure will be 160, 170, 180, or even over 200. On the bottom side of the pressure curve the opposite will happen. The arteries cannot constrict between beats; the pressure falls sharply. The diastolic pressure in such a case will be 60 or 50 or even lower. The difference between the systolic pressure and the diastolic pressure thus increases, or as a physician would put it, "the pulse pressure widens." The pulse pressure refers to the difference between the systolic and diastolic pressures. This kind of high blood pressure is not very dangerous and rarely causes anything except minor symptoms. If the systolic pressure rises much above 200, some medical attention may be necessary for the dizziness or headaches that can annoy the patient. Mild therapy of a medical nature can often reduce the systolic pressure and relieve the symptoms. The physician would call this **benign arteriosclerotic hypertension.** In other words, the patient has a relatively harmless form of high blood pressure caused by generalized hardening of the arteries.

However, systolic hypertension is not entirely harmless. Recent studies have shown that simple elevation of systolic pressure alone can produce cardiac complications because this kind of elevation increases the workload of the heart and may predispose it congestive heart failure or to various acute ischemic episodes in the myocardium—angina pectoris or myocardial infarction.

Diastolic hypertension

In the relatively mild type of hypertension caused by hardening of the larger arteries only the systolic pressure rises. The diastolic pressure falls. When *both* the systolic and diastolic pressures rise, a much more serious disease is present (Fig. 8-2). "Diastolic hypertension" describes this kind of elevated blood pressure. It means that the diastolic pressure rises together with the systolic pres-

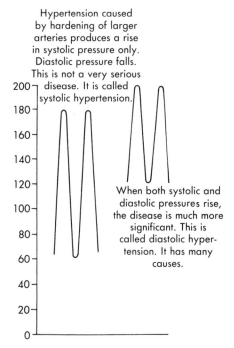

Hypertension caused
by hardening of larger
arteries produces a rise
in systolic pressure only.
Diastolic pressure falls.
This is not a very serious
disease. It is called
systolic hypertension.

When both systolic and
diastolic pressures rise,
the disease is much more
significant. This is
called diastolic hyper-
tension. It has many
causes.

Fig. 8-2. Hypertension. Hypertensive levels of blood pressure.

sure. The beast that threatens the patient now is a different creature and may be a very dangerous one. There are many kinds and degrees of diastolic hypertension; some are extremely mild and easily controlled, and some are very severe and can be a very serious threat to life or to health.

A serious rise in both systolic and diastolic pressures such as a figure of 220/130 is dangerous for several reasons. First, it puts a load on the left ventricle that must pump against increased pressure. Imagine that a man had been pumping water up a two-story building all his life. Then imagine that he was suddenly asked to pump the same amount of water every day up a ten-story building. Two things would happen: at the start, the man would work mightily and would grow very impressive muscles in the process, then he would begin to fail because he was exhausted; at last he would stop pumping altogether because he simply could not go on or because he had died of fatigue.

When the left ventricle pumps against an abnormally high blood pressure for a long time, the heart muscle becomes tremendously thickened. If the blood pressure is not lowered by medical measures, the heart muscle may fail, and the sequence of congestive heart failure, or left heart failure, begins. Diastolic hypertension also puts a dangerous strain on the wall of the arteries, just as if a tire were overinflated for a long period of time. This often leads to a rupture of any of the small arteries in the brain, producing what is called a **stroke**.

Finally, a very high blood pressure appears to affect the kidneys. A "chicken-and-egg" argument goes on here. It is clear that some kinds of kidney disease can cause high blood pressure. It is thought that some kinds of high blood pressure can harm the kidneys. The question of which comes first is not always clear, but there is no question that kidney disease of a very serious kind is often associated with prolonged elevation of blood pressure.

Causes of diastolic hypertension

Essential hypertension. The word "essential" reminds me of some high-ranking military figures I encountered during World War II. It is an impressive, mysterious term with almost no significance. When a physician calls a disease essential, he means that he does not know the cause. If a patient had a high fever for no known cause, the diagnosis of "essential hyperpyrexia" would be a lovely smoke screen for medical ignorance.

Unfortunately, many cases of diastolic hypertension fall into the class of "essential," meaning that the cause is not known. A man of middle age may find that his pressure has suddenly risen to 180/120 or some such figure. The physician examines him thoroughly, checking for kidney disease, growth in the adrenal glands, and all other factors that may contribute to blood pressure rise, but finds nothing. The case is then classed as essential hypertension.

Essential diastolic hypertension may be so mild that it is never any more than a minor nuisance. The blood pressure, for example, might rise to 160/100 or 170/100 in times of crisis or emotional tension, only to fall to normal levels with proper management, including rest. On the other hand, some types of essential hypertension may be very troubling and dangerous. The pressure may rise to figures like 210/120 and may stay there for long periods. This kind of prolonged elevated pressure exposes the patient to the two dangers of overloading the left ventricle with consequent congestive heart failure or rupture of an artery in the brain and death of brain tissue (in other words, a stroke).

The medical profession does not feel happy about using the word "essential" in describing any disease. Researchers have put staggering effort into attempts to run down the cause or causes of this kind of elevation of blood pressure. So far they haven't been very successful, but a few leads seem promising. Some workers believe that some type of kidney disease, which at this point lies beyond our methods of detection, may produce much of this kind of hypertension. Studies in this direction are certainly promising.

Certain nerves are also involved in essential hypertension. Nerves that run from nerve ganglia in front of the spinal vertebrae in the chest out to the blood vessels of the internal organs are thought to be involved. These are called the **sympathetic** nerves. Stimulation of these nerves causes a rise in blood pressure; in some patients this kind of stimulation through the sympathetic nervous system may be a large factor in development of essential diastolic hypertension.

In the past the sympathetic nerves were often cut in an attempt to control hypertension. This procedure has been discarded since the risk is high, the fall in blood pressure temporary, and the results poorer than those that can be obtained with medical management.

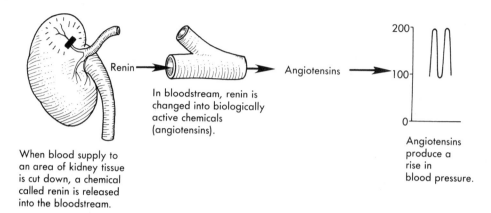

Renin

In bloodstream, renin is changed into biologically active chemicals (angiotensins).

Angiotensins

When blood supply to an area of kidney tissue is cut down, a chemical called renin is released into the bloodstream.

Angiotensins produce a rise in blood pressure.

Fig. 8-3. Cause of renal hypertension (elevated blood pressure associated with kidney disease).

Essential hypertension is probably a complex phenomenon, the result of the interplay of many factors—the resistance of the blood vessels to the passage of blood, the balance of salt and water in the body, certain endocrine factors, and, certainly, an inherited predisposition.

The kidneys and high blood pressure. An experiment carried out by Dr. Goldblatt opened the door to our modern understanding of high blood pressure and its relationship to kidney disease. Dr. Goldblatt clamped the artery leading to one kidney in a dog. He clamped it so that the blood flow to that kidney was cut down significantly. When this happened, the blood pressure rose and remained elevated as long as the blood flow was diminished. This was a classic experiment; it opened the door to a tremendous amount of research into the causes of hypertension.

Why does reducing blood flow to kidney tissues produce a rise in blood pressure? The answers to this question have been hammered out in research laboratories all over the world. Kidney tissue that does not have an adequate blood supply releases a large quantity of a substance called renin into the bloodstream (Fig. 8-3). Renin reacts with a certain protein in the blood to make yet another chemical called angiotensin. There are at least two forms of angiotensin; the angiotensins have the immediate, powerful effect of raising the blood pressure.

This kind of reduced blood flow can be caused by many kinds of kidney disease. Large stones in the kidney that compress the tissue can cut down blood flow enough to cause a rise in blood pressure. Chronic infection in the kidneys can do the same thing. Hardening of the arteries in the kidney or blood clots in arteries in the kidney again can produce the renin-angiotensin–high blood pressure chain reaction. Chronic inflammation such as Bright's disease results in a scarred set of kidneys with much inadequate blood flow and a rise in blood pressure.

How often is this type of kidney disease the cause of diastolic hypertension? Physicians still argue the point, but with more sensitive methods of investigation of the kidneys it seems that the renin-angiotensin chain is the culprit in an ever larger percentage of cases. X-ray films of the blood vessels leading into the kidneys and scanning the kidney tissue with radioactive isotopes are two of the methods in common use that sometimes provide lifesaving information. They enable the physician to detect the diseased kidney tissue in time to begin surgical correction, often with complete control of the high blood pressure.

A "chicken-and-egg" argument goes on in this field as well. A man with very serious elevation of blood pressure is found to have hardening of the arteries in his kidneys with much damage to kidney tissues as a result. Was the hardening of the arteries the original disease? Was this a disease of the arteries all over the body that happened to involve the kidneys? Did the hardening of the arteries take place first in the kidneys and then by release of angiotensin cause the high blood pressure with further blood vessel damage? The answers to these and related questions lie in the future.

In summary, you should remember that many kinds of kidney disease can produce high blood pressure. These diseases have one thing in common—some kidney tissue, because of the disease, does not have an adequate blood supply. When the blood flow to kidney tissue is cut below a certain point, toxic substances are released into the bloodstream and a rise in blood pressure follows.

Pheochromocytoma

Pheochromocytoma is a rare but fascinating kind of high blood pressure. Fortunately, it is curable.

The adrenal glands are tiny structures that lie above each kidney. They produce vital chemicals that circulate in the body, of which epinephrine (adrenaline) and cortisone are probably the two best known. Epinephrine causes blood pressure to rise; this is an old, well-known phenomenon. If a physician fears that a patient's blood pressure is dropping below the danger point in certain kinds of shock, he administers epinephrine by injection, which often produces a dramatic rise in the blood pressure. This is one of the normal roles of epinephrine as it circulates in the body. On rare occasions a tumor may grow in the adrenal gland. This tumor may form tremendous quantities of epinephrine and flood the bloodstream with them periodically. When this happens, the blood pressure will rise fantastically, and the patient will notice symptoms such as dizziness, pounding headache, and shortness of breath. The pressure may rise, for example, from a normal of 118/78 to 220/140 in a matter of seconds. Certain specific tests are now available that make it possible to detect this kind of tumor with very great accuracy. Once it has been detected, the elevated blood pressure is cured by surgical removal of the tumor. The operation has become much safer than it was a few years ago because of a major advance in pharmacology: the introduction of nerve-blocking drugs makes it possible to neutralize the effects of the epinephrine-producing tumor prior to surgery. Formerly the hazard of strokes and related complications during and after removal of such a tumor was very great. Now the operation is quite safe, and when the postoperative period is past, the person is free of high blood pressure for life.

Adrenocortical adenomas

Other types of benign (noncancerous) growths in the outside, or cortex, of the adrenal gland may cause high blood pressure. These tumors manufacture a specific hormone that causes the body to retain an abnormal amount of salt and water, and sustained hypertension results. The research that identified these **aldosterone-producing tumors** was a genuine breakthrough in the field of hypertension. Surgery on the adrenal glands is not easy and should only be undertaken by a surgeon of exceptional and specific competence, but a significant number of cases of severe hypertension have been controlled following removal of these growths.

Hypertension of pregnancy

It has been estimated that over a quarter of a million women in the United States develop hypertension during pregnancy every year; a significant number of fetal deaths are caused by this hypertension. This is particularly unfortunate because the hypertension of pregnancy is relatively easy to treat.

Hypertension of pregnancy falls into one of two classes as follows:
1. Preeclampsia and eclampsia. This means high blood pressure plus evidence of kidney abnormality manifested by protein in the urine and retention of water, producing edema. If eclampsia is allowed to go untreated it can be very dangerous with convulsions and considerable hazard to the life of both the mother and the baby.
2. Essential hypertension associated with pregnancy. Many women who have preexisting essential hypertension will undergo a rise in pressure, particularly in the last few months of pregnancy. Sometimes essential hypertension and preeclampsia are combined with considerable risk to the fetus.

Cushing's syndrome

This is a relatively rare but dangerous cause of hypertension. The usual cause is overactivity of the pituitary gland in the base of the brain. The pituitary gland as the master gland of the endocrine system controls the activity of all the other endocrine glands; that is, the thyroids, parathyroids, pancreas, adrenals, and the sex glands. For reasons not well understood, in Cushing's syndrome the pituitary gland suddenly begins driving the adrenal glands at an abnormally high functional rate; the adrenal glands in turn produce the hypertension-generating hormones previously mentioned, and the blood pressure can become dangerously elevated. Sometimes this same syndrome results from simple adrenal overactivity because of a primary adrenal tumor without pituitary involvement.

For whichever cause, a severe rise in blood pressure in an obese patient with thin skin, muscle weakness, and loss of calcium from bones always raises suspicion of this particular syndrome. Sometimes complete surgical correction is possible.

• • •

Why should hypertension be treated? What is the risk if the blood pressure remains high? These are extremely important questions any person with hypertension has to answer because treatment of significant hypertension usually involves a lifetime of changed habits and in many cases the uses of various drugs.

To justify all this effort the hypertensive patient must have the answers to two questions. (1) What are the risks and complications of uncontrolled hypertension? (2) Does controlling hypertension prevent these complications?

COMPLICATIONS

The complications of hypertension are (1) heart disease, (2) stroke, (3) kidney failure, and (4) hypertensive crisis.

Cardiac complications of hypertension

One of the commonest causes of left heart failure as described in Chapter 3 is hypertension. When the left ventricle must pump against an abnormally high fluid pressure, the ventricle will first respond by thickening the muscle wall to pump more efficiently, but ultimately the ventricle will simply "wear out," and the deadly process of congestion of the lungs and left heart failure begins. In many surveys over 50% of all cases of congestive heart failure in large populations have been shown to be due to hypertension and hypertensive heart disease.

Coronary artery disease

Hypertension is a well-documented "risk factor" for coronary artery disease. Patients with uncontrolled high blood pressure are at least twice as likely to have coronary artery disease and coronary artery death as those with normal blood pressures other factors being equal. Hypertension increases the process of hardening in the coronary arteries, or atherosclerosis, simply because of the effect of the heightened pressure within the vessels themselves. In addition, the load imposed on the left ventricular muscle by the abnormally high pressure against which it pumps leads to increased demands for oxygen by the heart muscle. The combination of diminished supply through diseased vessels and increased need by the heart muscle is extremely dangerous and, in fact, is often lethal.

Dissecting aneurysm

Fortunately, dissecting aneurysm is a relatively rare complication of hypertension, but when it occurs it constitutes an emergency. Sometimes the lining of the aorta actually rips or tears horizontally just past the origin of this vessel from the heart. The small tear may be produced by structural weakness in the wall of the aorta itself or in some cases it may be produced by a "ripping" action of blood moving under very high pressure and exerting great lateral forces against the wall. The tear goes part way through the wall but not completely. Once the smooth inside surface of the great artery has torn, blood forces its way between the coats of the vessel and "dissects" its way along, actually tearing the vessel as if one ran a knife between two layers of tissue, dissecting them apart. This mass of dissecting blood may work its way all around the arch of the aorta and down into the part of the vessel that leads to the abdomen. Sometimes the aortic valve is involved. Aortic dissection is, of course, an emergency, but with prompt medical and surgical intervention survival is the rule.

Strokes

The word "stroke" means a sudden interruption of blood flow to some part of the brain. The commonest cause of a stroke is rupture of a blood vessel or plugging of a blood vessel by an atheroma similar to the atheromas that form in the coronary arteries. Hypertension is by far the commonest cause of this kind of catastrophe; it is estimated that it occurs at least twenty times as commonly in patients with hypertension as in those with normal blood pressures.

Kidney failure

Again we confront the "chicken and egg." Progressive failure of the kidneys is extremely common in patients with uncontrolled hypertension. It is not clear whether the kidney disease really produces the hypertension or vice versa, but there is no question that the two are linked.

Hypertensive crisis

Any kind of hypertension may produce a hypertensive crisis; every patient with hypertension should be familiar with this syndrome and with its significance.

For any of a number of reasons the blood pressure may rise suddenly and dangerously; a patient with mild hypertension in the range of 150/90 may suddenly have a rise in pressure to levels like 280/150. At this time there will always be symptoms, and there is great danger. The patient will almost invariably describe some symptoms referable to the central nervous system; that is, headache, seizures, disturbances of vision, or actual unconsciousness. The sudden load on the heart may bring on severe worsening of chronic angina pectoris or may produce abrupt congestive heart failure. The kidneys may be affected with complete shutdown of urine production and failure of processing of the waste products of protein metabolism with consequent uremic poisoning. A hypertensive crisis is a life-threatening emergency that calls for immediate vigorous medical intervention; it can with proper therapy practically always be controlled.

TREATMENT OF HYPERTENSION

Every hypertensive patient should insist on a program of treatment that has as its goal the restoration of normal blood pressure levels. Treatment of hypertension is a lifelong commitment; it involves changes of habits and activities and a great deal of manipulation of powerful drugs, but this particular game is worth any candle.

Reducing blood pressure to normal levels and keeping it there completely eradicates some of the complications of hypertension and greatly reduces the risk of others.

For years physicians argued about the benefits of controlling hypertension; they asked whether lowering blood pressure really protected against strokes and cardiovascular complications. Large-scale studies in the past ten years have left no doubt in any responsible medical mind about the answer to that question.

Control of hypertension reduces the risk of myocardial infarction and coronary death by at least 50%.

Complete return of high blood pressure to normal levels comes close to eradicating the increased risk of strokes and kidney complications as well as of hypertensive crises.

Successful and sustained treatment of hypertension is quite literally a life-and-death affair.

Types of treatment

Today practically all hypertension can be controlled; the blood pressure can be brought to normal or near-normal levels and can be kept there. This is a revolutionary advance in preventive cardiology; it is probably more important in terms of total human benefit than all the brilliant technology of coronary bypass surgery.

Sodium (salt) restriction

A diet that is very low in sodium, the element that makes up about half of ordinary table salt, has been found to be helpful in most kinds of hypertension. Sodium restriction is really the basis for the so-called "rice diet" popular in the period immediately after World War II. If an individual's intake of sodium is very severely restricted—to about 200 milligrams per day—a surprising drop in blood pressure often takes place. The "rice diet," or "200 milligram sodium diet," is extremely severe; ordinary milk and various foods that contain any significant quantity of salt cannot be used at all. Before modern drug therapy was available, however, these severe diets were surprisingly effective and certainly saved many lives.

Newer data suggest that even modest salt restriction is helpful in control of high blood pressure. The patient can take some simple measures; that is, avoiding any added salt in cooking or at the table, avoiding foods that contain a large amount of natural salt such as milk, cheese, and the like, avoiding processed foods that contain large amounts of sodium, and being on the lookout for excess sodium in artificially flavored drinks, medicines, etc.

Recent studies of remote South American Indian tribes who never use salt revealed that these fortunate abstainers never have high blood pressure. Preliminary studies of schoolchildren and other population groups in the United States suggest that a lifelong low-sodium and high-potassium diet may actually prevent a great deal of hypertension. Although these studies are not complete, they suggest an exciting possibility—the mass prevention of hypertension and the complications that accompany it.

Obesity

Obese patients are about ten times as likely to have elevated blood pressures as their brethren. Every experienced physician has known for years that lowering weight in an obese hypertensive patient lowers the blood pressure, but nobody to this day can explain why. Nevertheless, there is no question that even with the beginnings of significant weight loss, that is, in the range of 10 or 20 pounds, the blood pressure will fall significantly and will continue to fall as the weight is lost. Even though the mechanism of this effect is not understood, it is so well-established that an extremely vigorous program of weight reduction is essential for the successful treatment of the obese hypertensive.

Drugs

When the rauwolfia drugs were introduced in the 1940s, the first forward stride in drug treatment of high blood pressure had been made. Various extracts of the plant *Rauwolfia serpentina,* an herb used for centuries by Hindu physicians, were found to drop the blood pressure in a surprising percentage of patients. A number of purified preparations came on the market, and the drug today is in wide and standard use. This is a mild form of treatment, but many physicians have had excellent results using the various extracts of this herb as a starting point for drug treatment in some forms of diastolic hypertension. There are serious side effects with rauwolfia, chief among them being ulcers in the stomach or duodenum. Some toxic mental effects have also been reported. In other words, like any other potent substance in medicine *Rauwolfia serpentina* can be harmful as well as helpful; it has to be taken under careful supervision.

Certain nerve-blocking drugs known as ganglionic blockers came into use in the early 1950s. These are still used in some cases of severe high blood pressure in which other agents do not control the disease. Again, they have some unfortunate side effects; these drugs drop the blood pressure so sharply that the patient may faint when he stands up or moves about. In some cases, however, under the supervision of a competent, skilled physician these drugs are still very useful and often give the physician a kind of "ultimate weapon" for the severe, difficult case.

The chlorothiazide group of drugs appeared somewhat later; these have been tremendously helpful in several fields of cardiovascular treatment. Chlorothiazide is a long-acting substance that pulls the sodium out of the tissues and causes it to move out through the kidneys in the urine. By doing this the drug puts the patient on a low-sodium diet automatically. This is so effective in many cases of high blood pressure that a great many physicians start with this drug as their first step in treatment of hypertension. If this does not control the pressure adequately, they will then add a rauwolfia preparation, still keeping up the chlorothiazide treatment. Chlorothiazide, too, has side effects that may be dangerous; for example, the mineral element potassium is pulled out of the tissues together with the sodium, sometimes to a threatening degree. Physicians had to learn by experience that patients who take chlorothiozide drugs must often have extra potassium, either in the form of special foods or as medication to replace the loss that almost certainly comes with the use of these drugs. When the potassium level drops too low, certain abnormalities of the heartbeat may follow, with very serious consequences.

Other diuretic drugs are now available, so that the physician has a choice of quick-acting or slow-acting diuretics or of diuretics that may be effective when the chlorothiazides fail.

Generally, a diuretic drug, often with some dietary restrictions, will be the first line of treatment, and alone will often control hypertension. If this is not sufficient, the physician may proceed to "second-line" drugs, which will include reserpine, alphamethyldopa, propanolol, or clonidine. These have varying kinds of action, but they are all powerful antihypertensive agents, each with significant side effects. Careful supervision is essential while the patient is being stabilized.

"Third-line" drugs will include agents that dilate blood vessels, thus lowering blood pressure—prazosine, hydralazine, and nitroprusside are the three principal useful drugs in this category.

The beta-blocking drugs used in the treatment of angina pectoris are very useful in the management of hypertension. Propranolol alone or in combination with other drugs has proved extremely effective and sometimes is the single critical element in a program of antihypertensive therapy.

Very powerful nerve-blocking drugs are available to resistant cases, but are rarely used at this time because of the availability of better and safer drugs.

For treatment of hypertensive crisis when the brain is acutely "water-logged" and small blood clots and areas of hemorrhage form within the brain tissues, rapidly acting drugs such as diazoxide and nitroprusside, which can be used intravenously, are often lifesaving. Management of hypertensive crisis requires considerable skill and judgment and frequently some specialized equipment. Patients who live in smaller communities would do well to discuss the availability of such equipment and procedures with their physicians.

It isn't necessary to try to memorize all these drugs and their advantages and disadvantages, but any patient with hypertension needs to remember three things.

First, drug therapy can now control the great majority of cases of high blood pressure. It is safe to say that over 80% of all patients can be held to normal blood pressure levels for many years. However, drug therapy is usually progressive in a stepwise fashion. This means that the physician will start with one drug such as chlorothiazide or rauwolfia and then if the blood pressure is not down far enough, add another, and then a third, and sometimes a fourth. The drug must be balanced against the individual's blood pressure and against the individual's sensitivities and reactions. These will be completely different in every patient. It will take quite a lot of time and careful controlled experimentation in most cases of severe high blood pressure to reach the right combination of drugs. The patient's needs may also vary from month to month or year to year, thus changing of doses and drugs may have to go on for a long time.

Second, every one of the drugs listed previously can cause serious toxicity. Every one of them has side effects that are dangerous and can even be fatal. They are not to be taken like candy nor are they to be taken for long periods without medical checkups. Ulcers, low blood potassium levels, and mental effects are only a few of the toxic reactions that will assail the patient who takes these drugs for long periods without adequate supervision.

Third, these drugs do not **cure** hypertension any more than insulin **cures** diabetes. They do control it, however, and this is a tremendous advance over the "Dark Ages" of hypertension fifteen or twenty years ago. The patient with significant diastolic hypertension for which no specific cause can be found is going to have to take medication for a long time, probably for the rest of his life. This means a lot of pill taking, with possible annoying side effects and many visits to a doctor's office. If all this seems burdensome, however, compare these minor irritations with the outlook in 1940, when the patient with significant hypertension could look forward to a stroke, heart failure, or kidney failure! One of three ends was written into his fate inexorably. By happy contrast, today the hypertensive patient can look forward to a reasonably normal, healthy life span. The possibility of controlled hypertension is one of the great triumphs of preventive cardiology.

QUESTIONS FOR THE PATIENT

1. Do I have systolic hypertension or diastolic hypertension?
2. Is the hypertension fixed; that is, is it there all the time or does it come and go?
3. What is the effect of exercise on my blood pressure?
4. Would you class my hypertension as severe, moderate or mild? On what basis?
5. Has my blood pressure responded adequately to medical management, and if not, what further steps should be taken?
6. Can you be sure that my high blood pressure is not caused by disease of the kidneys or the adrenal glands or possibly the arteries to the kidneys?
7. Do you detect any complications of high blood pressure in my heart, my brain, or my kidneys?

9   The heart valves: types of abnormal function; heart sounds and murmurs

The metal "flap" shown in Fig. 1-4 will not work forever; in some way it will finally begin to wear out. Remember this valve consists of two flaps of metal hinged so that they swing open and shut exactly like a pair of swinging doors. What could go wrong? The hinges might become rusty; masses of rust might clog the hinges so that the flaps could open only a little way (stenosis, Fig. 9-1, *B*). The fluid flowing through the pipe will now "back up" behind the partially stuck hinge.

This happens in the valves of the heart. Remember these valves are flaps of living tissue. Certain diseases may attack them so that the tissues that form them become inflamed and infected. When the inflammation or infection leaves, scar tissue forms just as it forms in the skin after a cut heals. This scar tissue forms "adhesions" across the valves, gluing them partly shut. The valve in the heart is now exactly like the valve in the pipe with rusty hinges; it cannot open to its full width. Sometimes the valve can open only a little, so that there is a very small hole for the blood to flow through. Rheumatic fever is the commonest disease that forms this kind of scar tissue and adhesions in the valves. Narrowing of this type is called **stenosis.** Medically the word "stenosis" refers to any structure that is abnormally narrowed. In the case of heart valves stenosis means that the valve opening at its maximum is much smaller than it ought to be because the valve flaps have been partially stuck together with scar tissue.

The other way a valve might wear out is that the edges of the flap might become worn and rusty where they meet. The valve is supposed to be watertight in the pipe and bloodtight in the heart, and if it is not to leak, the edges must meet very tightly, like a pair of tightly fitted double doors. If the tissues along the meeting edges become shriveled and warped by scar tissue, the valve edges will not meet when the valve swings shut. Fluid will flow back through the valve to the chamber it came from. Rheumatic fever, again, is the commonest disease that scars and distorts the meeting edges of the heart valves so that the blood leaks back into the chamber it has just left. The medical term for this kind of leaking is **regurgitation.**

Often a heart valve that is diseased will be both stenotic and regurgitant; that is, the valve will be so scarred that it cannot swing widely open, and its meeting edges will be so deformed that blood will leak back through it.

Figs. 9-1, *B,* and 9-2 show what happens behind a stenotic mitral valve. Normally the blood flows from the lungs to the left atrium and through the mitral valve to the left ventricle, whence it is pumped to the body. Suppose the valve can open only to a quarter or less of its normal width. Back pressure will build up in the left atrium. From this chamber the back pressure soon moves up the pulmo-

107

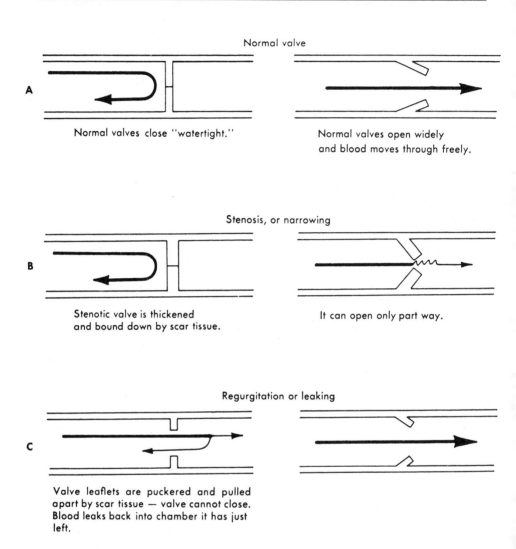

Fig. 9-1. Disease of the heart valves.

nary veins into the lungs. There will soon be an excess of blood in the lungs that cannot come out through the narrow mitral valve.

If the mitral valve leaks, the same thing happens, except that it usually does not happen as rapidly. Most of the blood will leave the left ventricle through the aorta to the body. If the mitral valve leaks, some of the blood that should go out through the aorta leaks back up through the diseased valve into the left atrium. When this goes on long enough, the same kind of back pressure will build up in the left atrium and thence back into the lungs.

Stenosis of the aortic valve may throw a severe load on the left ventricle. The great pumping chamber attempts to force a normal amount of blood out

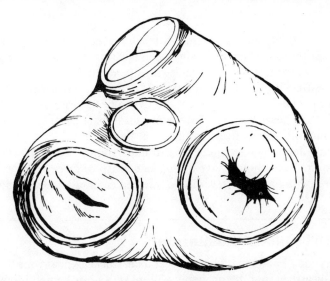

Fig. 9-2. Diseased heart valves. Left valve is stenotic. Valve flaps are bound together by masses of scar tissue. Note very small opening through which blood must flow. This is often called a "fish mouth" type valve. Right valve regurgitates, or leaks. Valve edges are shriveled and pulled apart by scar tissue—valve cannot swing shut. When ventricle below valve contracts, some blood will leak back into chamber it has left.

through a narrow opening. If this opening is very narrow, the muscle will be working against an impossible load. For a time the muscle will thicken as the heart tries to compensate to overcome this increased work load. Finally, the time will come when the back pressure in the left ventricle below the narrow valve will be too great, and the heart will begin to fail. The back pressure will then build up in the left atrium, into the lungs, and the same deadly chain of events will begin. Aortic stenosis has two other dangerous features. First, the amount of blood pumped out to the vital organs of the body diminishes sometimes past the danger point, and second, because of the type of blood flow leaving the aortic valve, the filling of the coronary arteries that feed the heart muscles is not very efficient. Leaking or regurgitation of the aortic valve throws a load on the left ventricle in a slightly different way. If a large volume of blood leaks back into the left ventricle after each contraction, the muscle finds itself working against odds. If a third of the blood pumped out leaks back, the muscle of the left ventricle, roughly speaking, must work a third harder than if the valve were healthy. Again, the muscle will finally wear out. First the muscle wall will thicken, and then the increased back pressure and volume of blood will balloon the ventricle out. When this happens, the heart is close to failure, and the same deadly chain of events is about to start. Increased pressure will back up into the lungs, and the patient will begin to notice that breathing is difficult.

Either stenosis or regurgitation of the valves of the left side of the heart will cause increased back pressure into the lungs and typical left heart failure.

The same things can happen to the valves of the right side of the heart, the pulmonic and tricuspid valves. Now all of the increased pressure will back up into the veins of the body, and the patient will have failure of the right heart with watery swelling of the tissues, or edema. The narrowing of a stenotic valve may be very slight. If the valve can still swing open 90% of the way, nothing much will happen to the patient; if the valve can swing open only 20% of the way, the heart will fail. The same is true of regurgitation. If a diseased valve leaks a few drops of blood with each heartbeat, the patient can live to be 95 years old and die of something other than heart disease; if the valve leaks back 30% or 40% of what is passed through it, serious heart trouble is at hand.

The reader should be quite sure to understand the terms "stenosis" and "regurgitation," and should have a thorough grasp of these terms as they apply to the valves of the heart. They will be referred to many times in this book.

Heart sounds and murmurs

Everybody knows that you can hear a heartbeat. Ask anyone to imitate the sound of a heartbeat and he probably will make a noise something like thump-bump, thump-bump; at any rate, he will make two sounds. Everyone has heard a rhythmic two-beat sound supposed to represent the sound of a beating heart on the radio, the television, or in assorted horror movies, and everyone remembers the telltale heart in Poe's tale, thumping away under the floorboards to the consternation of the maniac, but few people actually know what it is in the heart that produces the sounds of the heartbeat.

The heart sounds are produced by the slamming shut of the two sets of valves. The valves between the atria and the ventricles are the inlet valves to the ventricles. These are the atrioventricular valves—the tricuspid on the right and the mitral on the left. There is an outlet valve from each ventricle: the pulmonic valve allows the blood to run from the right ventricle out through the pulmonary artery; the aortic valve swings open to let the blood gush out to the aorta and the body from the left ventricle. The inlet valves swing open and shut at about the same time; so do the outlet valves. When these taut leaflets of living tissue swing together, the effect is the same as if one slammed shut a pair of double doors. Thudding vibrations are set up in the tissues around the valves with the production of a sound one can hear simply be putting the ear against the chest wall.

When the ventricles have filled with blood, the inlet valves swing shut, producing the first heart sound. After the ventricles have emptied their load of blood and are ready to start refilling, the outlet valves swing shut, producing the second heart sound.

The physician listening with a stethoscope will place the instrument on many areas of the chest because one hears the different sounds best in different places. Sometimes the two inlet valves close at exactly the same instant but most of the time they do not. There is usually a split-second difference between the closing of the mitral valve on the left and the tricuspid valve on the right. The mitral valve normally closes ahead of the tricuspid valve.

The same thing is true of the closing of the outlet valves; sometimes they close together, making a single sound, but more often the aortic valve closes a fraction of a second ahead of the pulmonic valve.

Physicians know more about listening to heart sounds now than they did ten or twenty years ago. Trained cardiologists can learn much about disease in the heart by noticing the splitting of sounds as one valve closes slightly ahead of the other. Certain types of splitting of sounds indicate heart disease and others are normal. Modern electronic recording devices have refined the physician's skills. A trained cardiologist can time the splitting of a heart sound within one- or two-hundredths of a second. This very tiny difference in time may be very important in making a diagnosis.

ORGANIC MURMURS

Now imagine that the valves are diseased; one can reason out the abnormal sounds that will follow. Suppose the aortic valve is scarred with rheumatic fever, so that the valve opening is only as big around as a ballpoint pen. The torrent of blood rushing through this narrow opening during systole will make a roaring sound, just as water makes a roaring noise going through a narrow, rocky passage in a river. This sound will begin immediately after the inlet valves have swung shut as the blood begins to flow out of the left ventricle into the aorta. In other words, it will start almost immediately after the first heart sound in most cases. When the blood has stopped rushing out through the narrow valve, the roaring noise will cease. There will be a brief moment of silence, and then the physician will hear the second heart sound. This is one kind of a **heart murmur.**

A heart murmur is a prolonged abnormal sound audible during some part of the heart cycle. It may be roaring or whispering, high-pitched and screeching, or soft and "blowing"; it may occur during systole or diastole; it may be short or prolonged. It may indicate serious heart disease, or it may have no significance at all (Fig. 9-3).

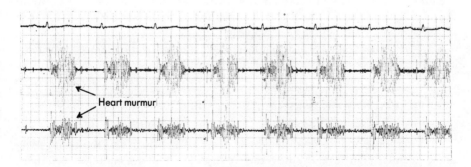

Heart murmur

Fig. 9-3. Phonocardiogram, or sound recording, of a heart murmur. The high-frequency vibrations indicated by arrows recorded at two different sound levels are a heart murmur. In this case the murmur is of aortic stenosis.

The roar of blood flowing through a narrow valve opening is only one kind of heart murmur. Suppose the mitral valve leaks with regurgitation of blood back into the left atrium when it should be going out through the aorta. Another prolonged abnormal noise will be caused by the flow of blood backward through the narrow opening of the leaking valve. This is a backward flow with different pressure characteristics and as a result the noise that it makes will be different. The physician can tell whether the murmur is caused by a backward flow through a leaking valve or a forward flow through a narrow valve by the pitch of the sound and by its duration. He will also notice whether the murmur lasts all the way from the first sound to the second sound and whether the murmur is of equal intensity all the way through systole.

These are two common types of heart murmur; there are hundreds more. If an aortic valve leaks blood back into the left ventricle during diastole when the ventricle is refilling, a murmur will come during diastole after the second heart sound. This again will have completey different characteristics of pitch and timing.

Heart murmurs produced by stenotic or regurgitant valves are possibly the most important murmurs the physician seeks; much time must be spent deciding how loud the murmur is, over what part of the chest it is heard, whether it is high or low in pitch, and where it comes in the heart cycle. Also it is important to know whether the murmur is associated with splitting of the valve sounds.

Some types of congenital heart disease produce murmurs. If there is a hole in the septum between the left and right sides of the heart, there will usually be a rush of blood through this hole at some time in the heart cycle. This will make still another kind of prolonged, abnormal noise, which may be high or low in pitch, short or long in duration, and occur at various times during the heart cycle.

The vegetations growing on the valves during bacterial endocarditis will of course produce swirling currents in the blood with a murmur that changes from day to day as the vegetations change in their shape and size. The physician will listen carefully every day for the changing murmur characteristic of bacterial endocarditis.

Other events in the heart can produce murmurs. If a patient has severe high blood pressure, the rush of blood from the left ventricle into the high-pressure area of the aorta will make a murmur because of the eddies and vibrations set up in the fluid mass of the blood. Certain disasters, such as a rupture of one of the tiny muscles that hold the heart valve in place or the perforation of the septum of the heart during a myocardial infarct, will produce very dramatic murmurs that one can sometimes hear without the stethoscope.

FUNCTIONAL MURMURS

The body responds to a number of conditions by increasing the volume of blood in response to increased metabolic needs of the tissues of the body: pregnancy, anemia, high fever, and overactive thyroid gland are common examples. There is nothing wrong with the heart itself, but because there is an unusually large amount of blood being pumped through it, murmurs will be generated. These murmurs are called **functional** murmurs. Hearing them, the physician will look for the cause of the increased blood volume rather than for disease of the heart.

INNOCENT MURMURS

Finally and most commonly, there is the innocent murmur. *Most prolonged abnormal sounds, or heart murmurs, do not mean anything. They are not the result of heart disease.* Practically everybody has some kind of murmur at some time in his life; innocent murmurs are particularly common in young people and adolescents.

These innocent, or harmless, murmurs are the result of eddies and whirlpools as the blood makes its swift, narrowed, tortuous way through the heart and lungs. Remember the blood must go around some pretty sharp corners as it moves through the chambers of the heart. Picture a river going around a sharp bend and you can imagine the eddies and whirlpools along the banks. If the banks of the river are really the walls of the heart, it is easy to imagine these high-frequency vibrations of the fluid creating abnormal sound. This is probably the common cause of the innocent, or harmless, murmurs. Millions of people have been told they have heart disease when they have not. The common reason for this is that the physician hears an innocent murmur and thinks that it is caused by disease in a valve.

• • •

On being informed that a murmur is present, therefore, the heart patient should logically ask three questions:
1. Is this an organic murmur? Is it caused by some structural abnormality in the heart valves, the great vessels, or the chambers of the heart?
2. Is it a functional murmur? Is it produced by some general abnormality of the body that demands an increased volume of blood, and if so, what is it?
3. Is it an innocent murmur? Can I safely ignore it?

A trained physician can tell a great deal about the health and disease of the heart by detecting abnormal sounds and murmurs. This is not easy, and not every physician can do it. The variety of heart murmurs, the location in the chest where they are heard, the differences in pitch, timing, and duration, together with the tiny differences in the splitting of the heart sounds add up to a vast and complicated subject. Whole textbooks have been written on the art of listening to the heart. The years of postgraduate training of a cardiologist include hundreds of hours of practice in the skills of cardiac physical examination; some of the cardiology fellows at our university center have commented to me that the process is like learning to play a complicated musical instrument by ear.

If a physician who is not a cardiologist asks for consultation in the assessment of abnormal heart sounds or murmurs, the patient should respect the physician's request and act on it. As a general rule the physician who is quick to ask for consultation is the physician who puts the patient's welfare first.

Advanced sound recording techniques are often used to make a permanent record of murmurs. Microphones are placed on the chest, and sometimes very tiny microphones are placed inside the heart itself through catheters moved in through the veins or arteries. This kind or recording is useful in a number of ways, but the chief usefulness of recording of heart sounds is that it trains the physician to hear more accurately.

The human ear is an incredible instrument; so is the human brain. When the two are combined with patient training and with the help of various electronic recording devices, the physician's ability to hear and to diagnose with a stethoscope may become fantastic. Medical science has ventured far into the fields of high fidelity only to make a better working instrument of the physician at the bedside with a stethoscope applied to the patient's chest.

QUESTIONS FOR THE PATIENT

If your physician tells you that you have a heart murmur:

1. Is this an innocent murmur? Can I disregard it?
2. Is it a functional murmur? Is it a result of increased blood flow, and if so, what's the cause?
3. Is my murmur caused by a diseased heart valve? Which one?

If your physician tells you that you have aortic stenosis:

1. Is this significant aortic stenosis?
2. Is it producing symptoms; that is, dizziness, fainting, anginal pain, or shortness of breath? If it is producing symptoms, shouldn't I have something done about it? Tell me how I can be sure I have aortic stenosis and not some other valve lesion.

If your physician tells you that you have mitral stenosis:

1. Is this stenosis severe enough to cause symptoms? Is that why I'm short of breath? If the mitral stenosis is actually causing symptoms, shouldn't it be operated on?
2. What are the dangers of a blood clot in the left atrium?

If you have aortic or mitral insufficiency:

1. How severe is the insufficiency? Is it causing any symptoms?
2. Is there any reason to consider surgical replacement of the valve?

For any valve lesion:

1. Should I be on rheumatic fever prophylaxis? Should I be on endocarditis prophylaxis?
2. Is my heart murmur caused by a congenital heart lesion? If so, exactly what is it?

10 Valvular heart disease

A number of diseases and degenerations may affect the valves of the heart. Rheumatic fever (Chapter 11) was formerly the commonest cause of structural abnormality of the heart valves, but at this time it is likely that a number of congenital and degenerative diseases are more important statistically, at least in the United States. When a heart valve is significantly deformed so that it cannot function efficiently, an increased work load will be forced on the heart muscle in one or more chambers if an adequate volume of blood is to be propelled out to the body despite the inefficient valve.

AORTIC REGURGITATION (LEAKING)

Imagine the aortic valve leaking so that anywhere from 30% to 50% of the amount of blood ejected out into the aorta leaks back into the left ventricle during diastole, or filling. The left ventricle can compensate for this for a time by "stretching"; that is, by an elongation of the muscle fibers that make up the chamber so that the chamber itself becomes larger to handle this increased blood load. Remember that during diastolic filling there is a constant rush of blood from the lungs through the left atrium into the left ventricle, and when to this predictable volume is added the extra blood that has leaked back into the ventricle from the aorta, the chamber must accommodate a greatly increased quantity of blood. The heart being remarkably adaptable, the chamber can dilate, that is, passively distend, and the heart muscle can adapt itself to handle this increased load for some time. If the leak is very mild, the heart can accommodate the increased load throughout a normal life expectancy, but if the leak is severe, sooner or later the heart muscle is going to wear out. Ejection of blood from the left ventricle will become inefficient, the chamber will no longer be able to keep up with the volume of blood rushing in from the lungs with each beat, and the phenomenon of "back pressure" described in Chapter 3 will begin (Fig. 10-1).

Thus the effects of significant aortic regurgitation are as follows:
1. Enlargement of the left ventricular chamber with distention of the chamber by an increased volume of blood and thickening of the muscle wall as the muscle tries to accommodate the increased work load.
2. Congestive heart failure, sometimes accompanied by pain arising from the overworked heart muscle.

Symptoms of aortic regurgitation

The symptom will be principally shortness of breath—the one real symptom of left heart failure. The shortness of breath will be progressive, slowly or rapidly, depending on the severity of the leak, and in the terminal stages the patient is unable to do more than sit in a chair or rest in bed. *Orthopnea,* or shortness of breath noted when lying flat and relieved by sitting up, commonly occurring late at night, will develop in the moderate to advanced stages of the disease. Pain somewhat like the pain of coronary artery disease may be present particularly at night and may sometimes awaken the patient.

Diagnosis

It is easy to diagnose aortic regurgitation by the character of the pulses, the unusually wide pulse pressure; that is, the difference between the systolic and diastolic pressures, and by the characteristic murmur of aortic regurgitation heard with the stethoscope.

The difficult question is to decide how severe the aortic regurgitation is, and for this the physician must usually turn to diagnostic instruments, at least in the early stages of the disease. *Detection of left ventricular enlargement* by x-ray examination, by the electrocardiogram, or by the echocardiogram will be the physician's chief concern, in addition to a careful history, looking for symptoms suggestive of early congestive heart failure. An abnormally large diameter of the left ventricular chamber at the end of filling, or diastole, is probably the most important single measurement the cardiologist can make.

Treatment

In mild cases no treatment may be necessary except for endocarditis prophylaxis (Appendix 2). In mild to moderate cases the physician will customarily use the usual armament for congestive heart failure, including digitalis, diuretics, and more recently, vasodilators, that is, drugs which will "open up" the arteries of the body and make it easier for the blood to flow out into them. The more blood that flows out into the vessels of the body, the less will regurgitate into the left ventricle, generally speaking, and the use of vasodilator drugs has been dramatically helpful in cases of aortic regurgitation resistant to other forms of treatment.

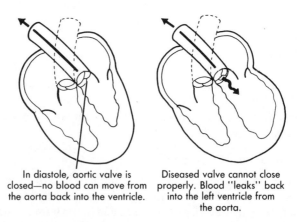

In diastole, aortic valve is closed—no blood can move from the aorta back into the ventricle.

Diseased valve cannot close properly. Blood "leaks" back into the left ventricle from the aorta.

Fig. 10-1. Effect of aortic regurgitation. Note leakage of a large volume of blood back into the left ventricle from the aorta.

Surgical replacement of the aortic valve may be the best way to treat symptomatic aortic regurgitation; this means that when the patient reports symptoms that are clearly caused by the regurgitant aortic valve, many physicians believe it is time to begin arrangements for surgery. All data accumulated in the last few years indicate that waiting too long can be very dangerous; up to a point the distended, thickened left ventricle can recover a good deal of its function and approach its normal size, but there is a very definite "point of no return." If the disease is allowed to progress too far, the left ventricle becomes irreversibly damaged and the patient will have serious problems even after surgical correction of the leak.

The risk of surgery varies from 5% to 10% in medical centers where well-trained teams of experienced personnel are on hand. The risk during and after surgery is directly proportional to the degree of damage inflicted on the left ventricle by the increased load of the leaking aortic valve; for this reason the conscientious cardiologist will go to great lengths to estimate left ventricular function in a patient with aortic regurgitation even before symptoms have appeared. If there is evidence of declining ventricular function or very significant increase in ventricular size, surgery may well be indicated even before the patient begins to notice it.

AORTIC STENOSIS

When the outlet between the left ventricle and the aorta is narrowed, the muscle of the left ventricle must work harder to push the blood through the abnormally small hole. Naturally, there is a high pressure in the ventricle (Fig. 10-2), just as there would be a high pressure in a pipe upstream from an area that had been partly plugged up or narrowed by some obstruction. In contrast to aortic regurgitation there is no increase in volume of blood in the left ventricle when aortic

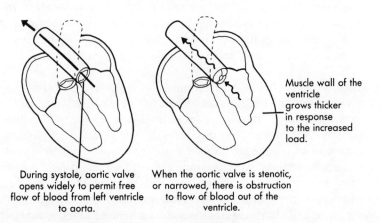

Muscle wall of the ventricle grows thicker in response to the increased load.

During systole, aortic valve opens widely to permit free flow of blood from left ventricle to aorta.

When the aortic valve is stenotic, or narrowed, there is obstruction to flow of blood out of the ventricle.

Fig. 10-2. Aortic stenosis. There is an obstruction to the flow of blood from the left ventricle out to the aorta because of narrowing at the valve.

stenosis is present. Instead there is an increase in pressure in the chamber as the heart muscle squeezes down with extra force to try to expel its load through the narrowed outlet. Like any muscle working against an unusually heavy load, the left ventricular muscle thickens and for a considerable period of time the extra contracting force of this muscle can make up for the obstruction to flow out through the valve.

The stenosis characteristically becomes more severe slowly over years as the valve becomes stiffer, the adhesions grow firmer, and the effective outlet from the left ventricle becomes smaller.

There will usually be a long period when the patient is tolerating this abnormality well, but sometime in middle life, that is, in the 40s, 50s, or 60s, the symptoms of aortic stenosis will appear. At this point the patient is in great danger and surgery is practically always required.

The symptoms of aortic stenosis are therefore extremely important; recognizing them may quite literally be a life-and-death matter. They are as follows:

1. Angina pectoris. The patient may feel pain exactly like the pain of angina associated with disease in the coronary arteries. The difference is that with aortic stenosis the anginal pain is caused by the enormous thickening of the muscle wall of the left ventricle and the resulting great increase in need for coronary blood flow. Sooner or later the growth in muscle mass outstrips the blood supply and the patient will begin to feel typical discomfort on exertion and relief with rest.

2. Fainting or dizziness. Because of the reduced flow of blood out through the narrowed aortic valve, the patient will often have inadequate blood flow to the brain and will become very dizzy or will faint. This commonly happens on standing from a lying or sitting position; sometimes it is noted with exertion.

3. Left heart failure. The patient will notice increasing shortness of breath exactly as in any other kind of heart failure because of the inefficient expulsion of blood out through the diseased aortic valve and the subsequent "backing up" of pressure into the blood vessels of the lungs.

When any of these symptoms appear in a patient with aortic stenosis, there is a 50% risk of death within two years; medical measures will not accomplish anything significant, and surgery should be considered as soon as possible.

There are all degrees of aortic stenosis, of course; *mild* aortic stenosis may be well tolerated and the patient may be able to live through a normal life expectancy with no difficulty. The physical examination is very helpful in determining that aortic stenosis is present, but it is not possible to state from physical examination alone how severe the stenosis is. Thus the proper diagnostic study of the patient with aortic stenosis *without* symptoms includes very careful assessment of the thickness of the left ventricular wall and the size of the left ventricular chamber among other things. X-ray examination, echocardiograms, nuclear medicine studies, and electrocardiograms will all be used to try to make this vital assessment.

MITRAL REGURGITATION

Mitral regurgitation, or leaking of blood from the left ventricle back into the left atrium (Fig. 10-3), has been the commonest form of rheumatic heart disease. Now that there is very little rheumatic heart disease, at least in the Western World, the commonest cause of mitral regurgitation is probably disease of the tendons and muscles that support the valve and hold the leaflets in place. Sometimes hardening, or calcification, of the valve and the ring of tissue around it can cause regurgitation.

Very much as in aortic regurgitation there is an increased volume of blood in the left ventricle, since a great deal of the blood in that chamber, instead of being ejected out of the body, simply goes "backward" up into the left atrium and then reenters the ventricle during the next filling period together with the usual volume of blood rushing in from the lungs. As much as half the volume of blood in the ventricle may actually be ejected backward to the left atrium instead of forward out the aorta.

For a time the heart will make up for this leak two ways. First, the left ventricle can expand, or dilate, to accommodate the increased volume of blood and the muscle of the left ventricle can increase the force of contraction to expel an adequate quantity for the needs of the body. Second, the left atrium itself can expand, or dilate, enormously, thus becoming a kind of reservoir, or storage chamber, for the blood leaking backward from the ventricle.

If the regurgitation is severe, however, sooner or later these compensatory mechanisms will fail, and the patient will begin to notice the characteristic signs of left heart failure.

Mild mitral regurgitation with a small volume of blood leaking back into

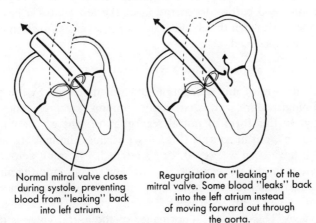

Normal mitral valve closes during systole, preventing blood from "leaking" back into left atrium.

Regurgitation or "leaking" of the mitral valve. Some blood "leaks" back into the left atrium instead of moving forward out through the aorta.

Fig. 10-3. Regurgitation or leakage of the mitral valve. A considerable volume of blood that should be ejected out through the aorta is leaking back up into the left atrium.

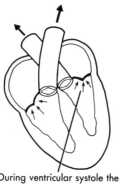 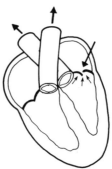

During ventricular systole the mitral valve must hold against a high pressure.

Sometimes one leaflet of the valve "gives" a little at peak pressure and "prolapses" or "lifts" a little into the atrium. This produces a characteristic set of sounds. The actual leak is insignificant and never leads to heart failure.

Fig. 10-4. Barlow's syndrome. Minimal leakage of the mitral valve because of weakened attachments. This is never a significant leak.

the left atrium is well tolerated and the patient may never need any medical management except for endocarditis prophylaxis. Moderate to severe mitral regurgitation can be managed for some time medically. Again, digitalis, diuretics, and in particular the vasodilator drugs that reduce the obstruction to the flow of blood out into the body have a very dramatic effect and may restore the patient to substantially normal function.

In the more severe forms of regurgitation surgery will be required; again, it is wise to intervene before degeneration of the left ventricle has passed the "point of no return" when the chamber cannot recover its function even though the leak has been corrected.

Mitral valve prolapse (Barlow's syndrome)

A special form of mitral regurgitation was described by the great South African cardiologist, Barlow; it is extremely common and rarely requires any vigorous therapy. In this form of mitral regurgitation, one of the mitral leaflets tends to "pop up" during systole (Fig. 10-4) because the tendons and muscles that support it have been weakened, or "stretched." A small amount of blood will regurgitate from the left ventricle into the left atrium, and the physician can hear a clicking sound when the valve pops upward into the atrium and often a short, late murmur as the blood rushes from the left ventricle through the weakened mitral valve. This type of abnormality of the mitral valve is often called "prolapse." Beyond endocarditis prophylaxis little is necessary in the way of medical management, and it is very rare for this kind of mitral disease to become so severe that surgery is needed.

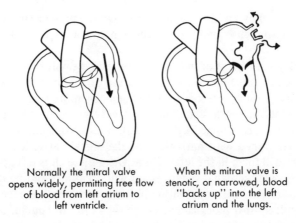

Normally the mitral valve opens widely, permitting free flow of blood from left atrium to left ventricle.

When the mitral valve is stenotic, or narrowed, blood "backs up" into the left atrium and the lungs.

Fig. 10-5. Mitral stenosis. Narrowing of the mitral valve hinders flow of blood from the lungs to the left ventricle.

MITRAL STENOSIS (Fig. 10-5)

Narrowing of the mitral valve is practically always caused by rheumatic heart disease. Unlike the valve abnormalities described so far, the left ventricle is not overloaded in mitral stenosis. On the contrary, there is a reduced volume of blood entering the left ventricle simply because the mitral valve, the orifice through which the blood flows from left atrium to left ventricle, is narrowed, sometimes to a small slit. There is back pressure above this narrow opening in the left atrium, and since there are no valves between the left atrium and the left ventricle, this increased pressure is quickly transmitted into the blood vessels of the lungs. Finally the increased pressure makes itself felt in the right ventricle, in the right atrium, and, as the disease progresses, in the veins of the whole body.

In other words, in mitral stenosis the blood "backs up" above the mitral valve in the left atrium and into the lungs. Naturally, the increased pressure of blood in the lungs quickly produces the classic manifestations of left heart failure; that is, shortness of breath on exertion, usually progressive, and orthopnea, severe shortness of breath coming on late at night. In addition, the high pressure in the small vessels of the lungs often causes blood to leak into the air spaces and be coughed up; a cough with bloody sputum is a classic finding in mitral stenosis.

As in the other valve diseases treatment depends on symptoms. Mild mitral stenosis with only slight narrowing of the valve orifice may be tolerated for life with no major medical measures needed. Once mitral stenosis becomes severe with progressive shortness of breath that limits that patient's activity significantly, surgery should always be considered because from this point on there is a very swift decline and relatively early death.

The one redeeming factor of mitral stenosis is that the left ventricle is not damaged as it is in mitral regurgitation or aortic valve disease. No matter how severe the mitral stenosis and no matter how high the pressure in the blood vessels of the lungs, the patient's symptoms will improve after the valve is opened or replaced.

Medical management of mitral stenosis relies heavily on the use of diuretics to drain extra water out through the kidneys and on digitalis to slow the heart rate when atrial fibrillation is present. In mitral stenosis more than in the other valve lesions blood clots in the left atrium are a very grave problem; patients with mitral stenosis are particularly likely to go into atrial fibrillation, and when this arrhythmia is combined with narrowing of the mitral valve, it is almost certain that blood clots will form in the left atrium. Once these clots have formed there is better than a 36% chance that one of them will break off and be discharged out into the body as an *embolus,* or floating blood clot, which will eventually plug up an artery someplace. If it blocks an artery to the brain, of course, the patient suffers a stroke, possibly with paralysis; blockage of arteries to the intestines, kidneys, other vital organs, or to the extremities can have very grave and sometimes catastrophic results.

In assessing the state of the patient with mitral stenosis, therefore, the physician will rely heavily on symptoms, on electrocardiographic evidence of enlargement of the left atrium or the right ventricle, and on the changes noted on the echocardiogram, which gives an excellent picture of the mitral valve itself.

PULMONIC STENOSIS

Stenosis of the pulmonic valve leading from right ventricle to pulmonary artery is practically always congenital. If the stenosis is severe the symptoms will be remarkably like those of aortic stenosis; that is, faintness of giddiness on exertion. When the pulmonic valve is narrowed, of course, a load is thrown on the right ventricle, which enlarges enormously. The only treatment for severe pulmonic stenosis is surgery, with simple cutting apart, or opening, of the adherent valve leaflets and relief of the stenosis. The results of surgery for pulmonic stenosis in skilled hands are excellent.

TRICUSPID DISEASE

Primary disease of the tricuspid valve is relatively rare; leaking of the tricuspid valve most commonly takes place because of back pressure caused by disease of the valves of the left side of the heart; that is, the aortic or mitral structures. Treatment directed primarily at the tricuspid valve is rarely necessary, but in some cases of congenital abnormality of the valve or of deformity of the valve as a result of endocarditis it is possible to correct a leak in the tricuspid valve surgically by simply reshaping the leaflets, stitching together lucent areas, and restoring the ability of the valve leaflets to close in a relatively watertight manner.

CARDIAC CATHETERIZATION

Before any patient with heart valve disease goes to surgery, cardiac catheterization (Fig. 10-6) will be essential to define the exact degree of valve abnor-

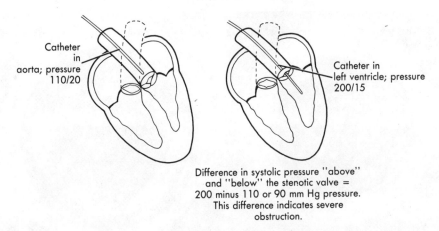

Catheter in aorta; pressure 110/20

Catheter in left ventricle; pressure 200/15

Difference in systolic pressure "above" and "below" the stenotic valve = 200 minus 110 or 90 mm Hg pressure. This difference indicates severe obstruction.

Fig. 10-6. Cardiac catheterization. The catheter is measuring pressures above and below the stenotic or narrowed valve to see how severe the narrowing is.

mality, guide the surgeon as to the exact measures that should be taken, and detect possible associated coronary artery disease. *The role of cardiac catheterization in valvular disease, therefore, is basically to determine how severe the lesion is.* The physician should be able to decide what valves are diseased and in what manner primarily by physical examination and what are called "noninvasive" measures—the electrocardiogram, x-ray examination, echocardiogram, and nuclear medicine studies.

During the catheterization the cardiologist will record the pressures above and below the diseased valve; if there is stenosis of the aortic valve, for example, there will be a very high pressure "upstream" from the narrowing and a relatively low pressure "downstream" from it. This difference in pressure is called a "gradient"; the size of the gradient is one of the most important considerations in deciding whether surgery is needed or not. In addition, by injecting dye into the chambers of the heart during catheterization it is possible to see regurgitation of blood from one chamber to another, for example, from left ventricle to left atrium when mitral regurgitation is present. By noticing the amount of dye moving backward, it is possible to estimate the severity of the regurgitation. Finally, it is possible to estimate ventricular function very accurately by measuring ventricular size at peak diameter in diastole and smallest diameter during systole. This can only be done, of course, when the ventricle is filled with dye injected through a catheter. The **ejection fraction,** or percentage of blood in the ventricle at the end of diastole that is ejected during systole, is the most important and most sensitive measurement of ventricular function. The ejection fraction enters largely into the surgeon's calculations about the safety of any proposed cardiac surgery.

PROSTHETIC HEART VALVES

Artificial heart valves may be either manufactured valves made out of plastic and steel or animal valves removed from a cow or a pig and specially preserved and supported for insertion into a human heart.

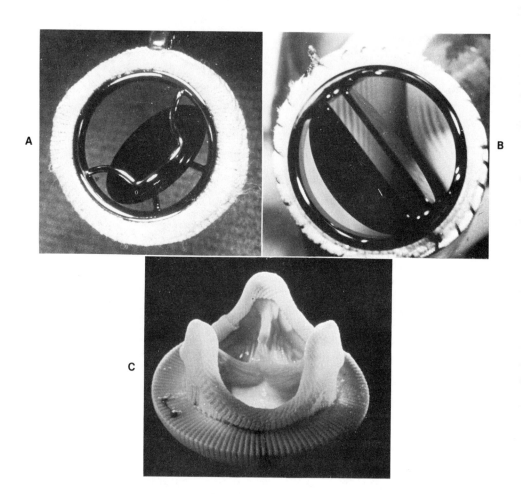

Fig. 10-7. A, Bjork-Shilly or tilting disc valve. **B,** St. Jude or double-flange valve. **C,** Hank-cock valve. A valve made out of an actual pig valve, often called a xenograft. (Courtesy of Dr. Richard Sanderson, Tuscon, Arizona.)

Several types of the plastic-and-steel valves are shown in Fig. 10-7, *A-C.* In general, these work either on a "flap" principle with a small disc opening and closing with the rush of blood or on a ball-valve principle with a tiny ball moving in a steel cage, also being propelled to and fro by the movement of blood during the heart cycle.

Any of these types of valves work quite well, but of course there are complications. Because these are mechanical devices, they can wear out; the steel or plastic parts can become deformed, and the valve can fail to function properly. Second, and much more important, blood clots may form on the valves, shutting them off entirely or reducing the amount of blood that can flow through them. Finally, infection, that is, endocarditis, can invade a prosthetic valve with the for-

mation of masses of infected clots on the valve structure or, much more dangerously, with abscesses in the ring where the valve is stitched into the heart.

Animal valves made from the actual heart valves of a cow or a pig work
very well for a time, but after some years these may undergo degeneration with
invasion of the valve tissue by hard, calcium-filled deposits and ultimate leaking
of the valve. These valves are much less susceptible to endocarditis and to clot
formation than the plastic-and-steel variety, but both complications certainly can
occur.

The important points for any patient with a prosthetic heart valve to remember are that (1) anticoagulant therapy is essential with any valve made of
foreign material such as plastic and steel; and (2) anticoagulation is essential with
animal valves in the mitral position. The question of whether anticoagulants
should be maintained when an animal aortic valve has been inserted is not yet ful-
ly resolved.

Endocarditis prevention is important with prosthetic valves. At the time of
any dental procedure, invasion of any body cavity that may be infected, childbirth, and the like, antibiotics should be prescribed in the usual manner (Appendix 2).

11 Rheumatic fever and rheumatic heart disease

RHEUMATIC FEVER

Until about twenty years ago most forms of valvular heart disease were the result of rheumatic fever and rheumatic heart disease. Today there has been a dramatic change. Rheumatic fever is becoming a very rare disease in the affluent nations of the Western World. In the underdeveloped nations of the Third World, on the other hand, rheumatic heart disease today remains the chief single cause of disability and death. In South America, Asia, and Africa rheumatic heart disease remains a major menace to life and health.

Rheumatic fever and rheumatic heart disease, while rare, have not completely disappeared from the United States; rheumatic heart disease continues to emerge in isolated and sporadic cases particularly among the poor and those isolated from modern medical care. There are some items of information about rheumatic fever and rheumatic heart disease that should be familiar to much of the general public especially to mothers of small children and to schoolteachers.

1. Rheumatic heart disease is the *only* completely preventable type of heart disease. It is *always* caused by rheumatic fever.
2. Rheumatic fever is *always* a result of an infection of the throat by a specific kind of bacteria—the group A beta-hemolytic *Streptococcus*. "Beta-hemolytic" refers to the action of this organism on the blood-agar plates used to grow it in the laboratory. This *Streptococcus* is the same type of bacteria that produces scarlet fever. To put it another way, the familiar "strep throat" is simply scarlet fever without a rash; scarlet fever is a "strep throat" with a rash. Except for the presence or absence of a skin rash, streptococcal pharyngitis and scarlet fever are identical diseases.
3. Rheumatic fever is classed as an *autoimmune* disease. In this type of disease the body generates antibodies to fight a particular infection—in this case the group A beta-hemolytic *Streptococcus*—but even after the bacteria have been eliminated, the protective immune reaction rages on, finally attacking the body's own cells, producing inflammation of the joints, brain, lungs, skin, and heart (Fig. 11-1). The situation is rather like the defenders of a fort who, having destroyed the invading enemy, go beserk and keep on shooting away the walls and supports of their own protective structure.
4. The streptococci that cause rheumatic fever are very easy to eliminate by antibiotic treatment; the difficult part is often diagnosis. Diagnosis of streptococcal infection of the throat can only be established by throat culture and bacteriologic study. A physician cannot tell by looking at a

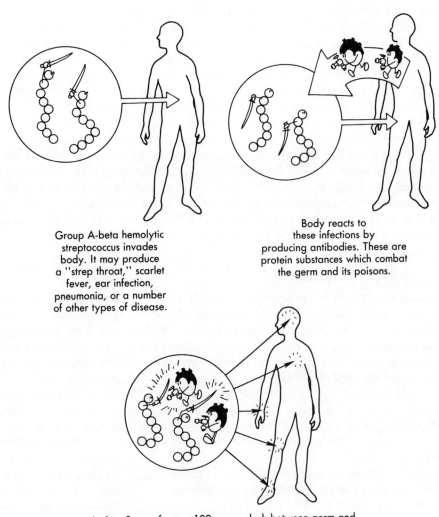

Group A-beta hemolytic streptococcus invades body. It may produce a "strep throat," scarlet fever, ear infection, pneumonia, or a number of other types of disease.

Body reacts to these infections by producing antibodies. These are protein substances which combat the germ and its poisons.

In 1 to 3 out of every 100 cases, clash between germ and antibodies starts a chain reaction of chronic inflammation in many areas of body. It attacks principally joints, heart, and brain. This chronic inflammation is called rheumatic fever.

Fig. 11-1. The reaction of rheumatic fever.

throat whether the inflammation is caused by streptococci or by some other type of organism such as a virus.

Clinical picture

Two or three weeks after a streptococcal infection of the throat the victim —usually a young person—may notice *soreness and swelling of the joints of the body.* This arthritis will move from one joint to another and will commonly involve several joints at a time. **Migratory polyarthritis,** to use the medical term, is the prime presenting symptom of acute rheumatic fever. The symptoms are produced by a self-perpetuating "chain reaction" in the connective tissues of the body characterized by a small inflammatory nodule rather like a group of pimples that have not quite come to a head and are so small they can be seen only with a microscope. These same inflammatory masses may involve the brain, producing St. Vitus dance; the lungs, where they produce pulmonary inflammation; the skin, where they form small, tender nodules; and most importantly, the heart.

If no treatment is administered, the symptoms of rheumatic fever may persist for some months before finally abating. The joints will not be permanently damaged, the irritation of the brain that produces the twitching motion of St. Vitus dance always disappears without any significant aftermath, and the pulmonary and skin complications never have any significant sequelae. It is the inflammation in the heart that is uniquely a hazard in rheumatic fever.

RHEUMATIC CARDITIS

All the layers of the heart may be inflamed in rheumatic carditis; that is, the pericardium, the epicardium, the heart muscle, or myocardium, and most importantly, the endocardium. In the acute stage of rheumatic fever coming on after an untreated streptococcal infection the whole heart may be reddened, swollen, inflamed, and very seriously weakened. The victim of acute rheumatic carditis may indeed die, and strenuous medical measures are frequently required.

After the acute inflammation has healed—and this may take weeks or months—a curious persistent process of inflammation and scarring with further inflammation and still further scarring goes on. This inflammatory-scarring process often involves the endocardium over the heart valves and the substance of the valves themselves so that the valves are distorted out of shape (Fig. 11-2). Sometimes the inflammatory spots which cluster along a valve edge will form "adhesions" between the valves, and they become stenotic. At other times the valves will be simply pulled apart by masses of scar tissue so that they cannot close when the valve swings together, and leaking regurgitation is the result.

Involvement of two valves is the rule in rheumatic carditis; the aortic and mitral valves are by far the most common targets of inflammation.

Diagnosis of rheumatic fever is sometimes very obvious, but sometimes it can confuse the most skilled clinician. Repeated blood tests to prove the presence of streptococcal infection, changes in the electrocardiogram, the appearance of certain specific types of heart murmurs, and the clinical characteristics of the migratory joint inflammation and other complications may all contribute toward establishing a definitive diagnosis.

Treatment may involve considerable periods of rest; aspirin is commonly employed in large doses. In severe cases steroids (drugs like cortisone) may be used to reduce inflammation, although there is no evidence that the use of these

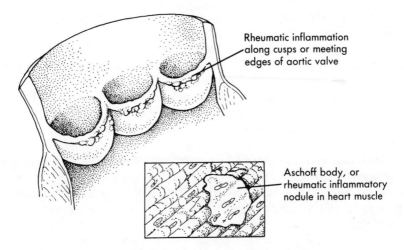

Rheumatic inflammation along cusps or meeting edges of aortic valve

Aschoff body, or rheumatic inflammatory nodule in heart muscle

Fig. 11-2. Rheumatic disease in heart valves.

drugs prevents the inflammation of the heart valves, which is the one really dreaded complication of rheumatic fever.

The extent of valve damage may not be clear at the time of the acute attack and, indeed, may not become clear for years after the event. In fact, once the rheumatic process has started, there is no really good treatment for rheumatic fever; the disease is going to run its course regardless of medical intervention.

Prevention of rheumatic carditis

Any reader concerned with rheumatic fever and rheumatic heart disease should underline the next three items of information: (1) The best thing to do about any disease is to prevent it; rheumatic fever and rheumatic heart disease are completely preventable. (2) Prevention is *everything* in rheumatic fever and rheumatic heart disease because once the disease is established, treatment is of little value. (3) Prevention of rheumatic fever and rheumatic heart disease is accomplished by detecting and treating group A beta-hemolytic streptococcal infections of the pharynx. Diagnosis of these infections can be ascertained only by throat culture and bacteriologic processing.

Prevention of first attacks

Since streptococcal pharyngitis can be identified and treated, why does rheumatic fever persist at all? There are several good reasons. In the first place a "strep throat" does not always follow the classic pattern of a severe sore throat with fever and swollen glands; in fact, serious streptococcal infections of the pharynx may be so mild the victim never brings it to anyone's attention, characterizing it as a "scratchy throat."

Second, physicians all too often neglect the vital step of taking a throat culture to detect the streptococci. As a further complication throat culture for streptococci usually cost too much ($5 to $10 or more).*

Third, parents all too often treat children's sore throats with lozenges, cough drops, or aspirin, none of which have the slightest effect in preventing rheumatic fever.

To take a throat culture on everyone in the whole country with a cold or sore throat would be an enormous expense; since rheumatic fever and rheumatic heart disease are very rare in most of the United States, the expense wouldn't be justified.

Detection and treatment of streptococcal disease should concentrate on groups at highest risk.

Rheumatic fever is a disease of the fall, winter, and spring months, primarily in children between the ages of 5 and 18. To put it another way, rheumatic fever and rheumatic heart disease are "occupational diseases of schoolchildren." This is true partly because youngsters seem to be more susceptible to the disease and partly because of the crowding inherent in any schoolroom.

Streptococcal detection and treatment therefore should concentrate on the following groups:

1. Schoolchildren.
2. Members of families with strong rheumatic fever histories or histories of repeated streptococcal infections. Many studies have shown that there is a genetic predisposition to streptococcal infection and its consequences in certain families.
3. Adults involved with large numbers of young children; for example, schoolteachers.
4. Families of children with repeated streptococcal infections who may harbor carriers. The term "carrier" refers to somebody with streptococci in the throat without symptoms or signs of inflammation. If the patient has a positive throat culture for streptococci, a physician cannot tell by looking at the throat whether an active infection is present or whether the person is in a carrier state. This differentiation can only be made by taking several blood determinations. (Again, in a low-risk group like the population of the United States, the distinction is not of great practical importance.)
5. Any patient of any age with a severe sore throat accompanied by fever, swollen glands, inflamed tonsils or purulent (pus-like) drainage in the throat should have a throat culture taken specifically for streptococcal detection.

Treatment

If a beta-hemolytic streptococcus infection of the pharynx is discovered, the patient should receive enough penicillin to provide an adequate blood level of

---

*The blood agar plates actually used to grow the bacteria cost about 25¢ and the other items used possibly a dime. Computing technicians' time and the cost of an office incubator, a throat culture for streptococci shouldn't cost more than $2 or $3, which still leaves some margin of profit for the physician or the laboratory.

the antibiotic for ten days. This level does not have to be very high, and it can be achieved by a simple shot of long-acting penicillin (benzathine penicillin). Oral penicillin will work just as well, but the tablets have to be taken three times a day for ten days, and it's very easy for patients to occasionally forget to take a tablet.

For patients who are allergic to penicillin, another antibiotic called erythromycin can be used. Again, the tablets should be taken daily for no less than ten days.

In a few "high-risk" areas of the country where streptococcal disease and rheumatic fever have been major public health problems, intensive programs to reduce streptococcal infection by mass screening of schoolchildren with enforced or free treatment of those found to harbor streptococci have been shown to be effective in reducing streptococcal levels and apparently in reducing or eradicating rheumatic fever and rheumatic heart disease. The possibility of this kind of mass control was first demonstrated by Rammelkamp and his colleagues at the Fort Warren Air Base in Cheyenne, Wyoming, during the Korean War, when that facility was almost closed by an outbreak of rheumatic fever. A program of intensive throat culturing and treatment halted the epidemic and permitted continued operation of the base. My colleagues and I applied the same principles in Casper, Wyoming, formerly a "high-risk" area, where a mass control project of throat culturing and treatment centered around schoolchildren and was extended through the rest of the population. The results in terms of control of streptococcal infection and apparent reduction in new cases of rheumatic fever were very gratifying and were used as models for similar programs in other areas. Today among the Papago and Navajo tribes of Arizona, in whom rheumatic heart disease was at least twenty to thirty times as prevalent as among the general United States population, mass control treatment programs have had very encouraging results. In the Papago tribe there have been no new cases for the past five years.

This kind of intensive surveillance and treatment, it should be emphasized, should be employed only in high-risk areas, but they may serve as a model for the Third World countries where the disease still rages largely unchecked.

Secondary prevention and treatment

Anyone who has had one attack of rheumatic fever has a 50-50 chance of having another. It is possible to prevent the "secondary" attacks with a high degree of efficiency, and "secondary prevention programs" are standard policy through most of the world today wherever economics and medical standards permit. Secondary prevention is based on keeping the streptococci out of the body; this is done by keeping an adequate level of antibiotic or sulfonamide circulating in the body continuously for years. *Streptococcus* never becomes resistant to penicillin, and hence this kind of prevention can be kept up through a whole lifetime. When this is done, the chance of a subsequent attack of rheumatic fever is greatly reduced, and the patient is given about 98% protection.

The standard recommendation is that any patient with a documented history of rheumatic fever be given intramuscular injections of long-acting (benzathine) penicillin at least until early adult life; some authorities recommend keeping up the injections "indefinitely."

The reason secondary prevention is important is that as far as anybody can tell, it is the recurrent attacks of rheumatic fever that "hammer away" at the heart valves, finally leaving the victim seriously incapacitated and possibly in danger of early death unless cardiac surgery corrects the abnormality. (A source of some confusion should be noted here; sulfonamide drugs should never be used for treatment of an established streptococcal infection because they do not prevent the subsequent development of rheumatic fever. On the other hand, in terms of secondary prevention sulfonamides are excellent for keeping streptococci out of the body; two tablets of sulfonamide a day can be used instead of the monthly shot of Bicillin.)

QUESTIONS FOR THE PATIENT

1. How do you know I have rheumatic fever?
2. Is there a rising antistreptococcal antibody titer (blood level of the body's natural defense substance specific to streptococci)?
3. Do I have polyarthritis; that is, swelling, pain, and tenderness in joints; or do I have polyarthralgia, simply a painful joint without any swelling or tenderness?
4. Is there evidence of rheumatic carditis—rheumatic inflammation of the heart? What is it?
5. How about secondary rheumatic fever prophylaxis from here on?

12 Pulmonary heart disease

Every reader of this book has seen somebody with chronic cor pulmonale, or pulmonary heart disease, and many of you actually have it. (Turn back to Fig. 3-2 to refresh your memory about right heart failure. Remember that *any* chronic disease in the lung may produce back pressure in the pulmonary artery and into the right heart. This increased pressure finally "backs up" through the veins of the body with watery swelling, or edema, in the tissues.)

Pulmonary heart disease is really a disease of the lungs, not the heart. You must remember sitting on a bus or subway across from some elderly gentleman who was obviously having a hard time breathing. If you had looked closely at him, you would have seen that his lips and earlobes had a peculiar bluish color. If you paid close attention, you would have noticed that it took him a long time to breathe out, or exhale—he seemed to breathe in normally but took a long time getting the air out again. You might also have noticed that as he walked to the door of the bus the effort made him gasp for breath and possibly halt midway down the aisle.

You were watching the most common cause of chronic pulmonary heart disease—chronic obstructive pulmonary disease, or COPD as it is commonly abbreviated. Sometimes the word "emphysema" is used to describe this syndrome, but, in fact, the lung disease is a mixture of chronic infection—bronchitis—and distention and rupture of the air cells—emphysema.

Our diseased bus rider might have behaved differently. He might have been coughing in spasms, making wheezing noises as he breathed in between the bouts of coughing. This would have been asthma with bronchitis, another common cause of chronic pulmonary heart disease.

If the bus happened to be in a hard-rock mining area, you would have seen many elderly men stopping to get their breath after they had walked up the steps onto the bus or after they had walked the length of the bus to their seats. You would have noticed that they sat and panted hard, as if they couldn't get very much air in and out of their lungs. The difficult breathing you would have seen would be different from the wheezing breathing of the man with asthmatic bronchitis or the forced, painful exhaling of the man with emphysema. These men would simply pant, like men who had walked up a steep hill. You would be looking at men with silicosis, another rather common form of chronic lung disease. Fortunately this disease is rarer than it used to be, but it still isn't rare enough.

This book is about heart disease, not lung disease; these disorders of the lungs are mentioned only as they affect the heart. Practically all chronic inflammations, infections, or degenerations in the lungs sooner or later produce a kind of resistance to the blood flowing into the lungs from the pulmonary artery. Scar tissue tends to compress the small vessels, and the whole effect on the blood flowing in from the right heart is much the same as if one tried to force blood through a system of pipes half plugged up with glue. Finally, the pressure in the pulmonary artery and its branches rises. Instead of a normal level of 10 or 12 millimeters of mercury, the systolic pressure may rise to 40, 60, 80, or even over 100 millimeters. Pulmonary hypertension, or high blood pressure in the pulmonary blood vessels, is now present. This is what the physician means by the term **cor pulmonale,** or pulmonary heart disease.

Treatment of pulmonary heart disease means treatment of the lung disease that causes it. Successful treatment of pulmonary heart disease means *early* diagnosis and treatment of lung disease before it goes past the point of no return. It means intelligent use of public health measures to prevent air pollution or exposure to toxic chemicals in industries. It means vigorous, continuing medical management of asthma with prompt treatment of the infections that always crop up during this disease. Hard-rock miners should work only in properly ventilated atmospheres or with proper filtration equipment worn when exposure to silica dust is necessary or unavoidable. Executives responsible for plants where workers will be exposed to fumes such as sulfur dioxide or will be inhaling particles such as asbestos have a very grave life-and-death responsibility to see that the atmosphere is as free as possible of these dangerous elements.

All these observations are important; they are also relatively minor. *The really major peril to the lungs of the American public is the inhalation of cigarette smoke many times per day.* There can be no question that in the patient with chronic bronchitis, asthmatic bronchitis, or emphysema, heavy smoking of cigarettes is a guarantee of chronic invalidism and early death.

Every major hospital holds large numbers of patients in the final stages of chronic cor pulmonale. They live in oxygen tents, gasping for breath, blue around the lips, earlobes, and fingernails, condemned to possible death and certain invalidism. The overwhelming majority of these tragic figures have been heavy cigarette smokers. It is odd that pipe or cigar smoking does not seem to be a serious factor in this type of lung disease. This is the same paradox that exists in the case of coronary artery disease and lung cancer. The answer, of course, lies in the depth to which the cigarette smoker inhales. Any confirmed cigarette smoker takes a deep "drag" and fills his lungs thoroughly with a cloud of toxins. The pipe or cigar smoker usually puffs in a superficial way, pulling a little smoke a short way down the windpipe or trachea, even though he will insist that he, too, "inhales."

The patient with chronic lung disease producing chronic cor pulmonale faces two disasters. He may die or at least become very ill from pulmonary failure as such, or he may die of right heart failure. Frequently he suffers from both.

Acute failure of the lungs, or acute pulmonary insufficiency, simply means that there is not sufficient oxygen moving through the alveolar membranes into the blood to feed the tissues. The word "acute" is a little misleading. Almost always these are people with chronic lung disease who have suddenly reached the "breaking point." There is simply not enough oxygen to feed the brain cells, for example, to maintain consciousness, and the patient sinks into a kind of coma. In 1950 patients rarely recovered from this kind of pulmonary failure. Today the picture is much brighter, although there is still a great deal of danger.

The physician treating this semiconscious, blue, obviously dying patient faces a problem. The patient needs oxygen desperately; in fact, he is dying for lack of it, but, on the other hand, if the physician simply gives oxygen in a mask, catheter, or tent, the patient may stop breathing entirely and die. This is the time when oxygen may actually be a deadly poison.

Why would this patient stop breathing and go into coma simply because oxygen was administered? The muscular act of breathing is controlled by a small area in the brain stem called the **breathing center.** This amazing mass of nerve tissue acts exactly the way a thermostat does in a house, except that instead of responding to changes in temperature, it responds to changes in the levels of oxygen and carbon dioxide in the blood. Remember that one inhales oxygen and blows out carbon dioxide. If breathing is inefficient, the carbon dioxide level in the blood rises very quickly while the oxygen level falls. In either case the patient will usually breathe more deeply and rapidly to correct the abnormality, that is, to take in more oxygen or blow out more carbon dioxide.

The patient with chronic lung disease has not been breathing out the carbon dioxide very well, and therefore there is a high level of carbon dioxide in his bloodstream all the time. If oxygen is administered, the breathing is likely to become less active as the blood oxygen begins to rise, and this sudden diminution in breathing activity will cause a catastrophic rise in the carbon dioxide level in the blood. The patient may then go into what is called carbon dioxide narcosis, go into coma, and even stop breathing entirely.

How does one get oxygen to the tissues? This can be done in one of several ways. In the great majority of cases the use of a low level of oxygen administered through a mask or nasal tube together with appropriate stimulants, both physical and medical, and treatment of the underlying disease with bronchodilators or antibiotics will correct the abnormality. Often, encouraging the patient to cough and breathe deeply is lifesaving. Hence trained nursing care makes the difference between success and failure.

For very severe cases the physician may put a tube into the trachea or windpipe and connect this tube to an automatic breathing apparatus that will breathe for the patient. Oxygen can now be pumped into the lungs in great quantities without any voluntary breathing effort on the patient's part at all. The "artificial lung" connected to the tracheostomy tube simply breathes for the patient until he is ready to take up the breathing himself.

The effect of these machines is often dramatic; but like most major medical interventions there may be complications. Profound changes take place in the body chemistry when this kind of aided breathing begins. The physician must be alert to these changes and must be ready to correct them with electrolytes (charged particles of potassium, sodium, etc.) and the like. Mechanically aided ventilation, properly performed, can produce very satisfying results—the patient who has been unconscious or semiconscious, blue, and possibly delirious or obviously near death, often turns a normal pink color in a matter of hours or even sooner. Frequently these patients fall into a healthy deep sleep because they have been almost exhausted by their struggles to breathe.

It should be emphasized that mechanically aided ventilation through a tracheostomy or endotracheal tube is a last resort, since it is sometimes very difficult to get a chronic lung patient "weaned" off this type of machine. Conservative measures are much more desirable when it is possible and safe to use them.

The brain may have been somewhat damaged by the prolonged period of low oxygen supply, and it may take days for the patient to return to anything like reasoning consciousness. Various heart medications may have to be used, including digitalis and diuretics.

In the great majority of cases of dangerous pulmonary failure the physician by one means or another can introduce enough oxygen into the tissues to maintain life, can correct abnormal mineral and chemical levels in the body, and can strengthen the heart and drain out edema fluid from the tissues. After some hours or days of intensive care in this manner the patient may be alert, breathing comfortably, and ready for the next step in rehabilitation directed to the chronic, severe pulmonary inadequacy.

Now the physician has many modes of attack; the choice depends on the basic disease present.

INFECTION

If a specific infection such as tuberculosis is present, the physician will treat it with specific drugs. Sometimes a great deal of study of the sputum will be necessary to find the kind of infecting bacteria present. Further studies will be necessary to find what antibiotics or chemicals will kill or slow the growth of the bacteria. One can sum up the treatment approach to chronic lung infection by saying that first a diagnosis is made by x-ray examination, by examination of the sputum, and sometimes by various skin tests. Then wherever possible the specific infection is attacked with antibiotics or chemicals. One of the great pillars on which the whole structure of treatment of chronic lung disease rests is *detection and treatment of infection, acute or chronic.*

OPENING OF AIRWAYS

Many victims of chronic cor pulmonale suffer from asthma; it is characteristic of asthma that the small airways tend to become congested and partly closed, very much like the nostrils during a bad cold. This partial plugging of the small airways is caused by two things; first, a great deal of mucus, or secretion, piles up, thereby plugging them up; second, there is often spasm, or squeezing down, of these small airways. To picture what the combination of these two factors can do, simply think of your nose when it is plugged completely shut by a bad cold. Various drugs are available that will open the airways and shrink the swollen, watery lining tissues. Adrenalin is the oldest and best known of these. Many synthetic substitutes have been invented, some of them with considerable advantages over Adrenalin. These bronchodilators, or "openers of the bronchioles," may be given by injection, in pill form, or, best of all, may be breathed with one of several machines directly into the lungs. If spasm of the airways is an important part of any chronic lung disease, the use of bronchodilators will be essential.

Inhalation therapy

Inhalation therapy is a prominent part of treatment for most kinds of chronic pulmonary failure. Various devices are available which produce a mist; bronchodilators and other medications can be suspended in this mist, which the patient inhales. In some cases it may be desirable to introduce this medication-laden mist under pressure with the hope that plugged or partly open smaller airways may be distended and reventilated. This kind of positive-pressure breathing is particularly useful after surgery when "it hurts too much to cough." Failure to cough adequately may produce inadequate ventilation of some parts of the lung with collapse of air cells, or atelectasis. Here the effect of the positive pressure in reinflating or reventilating the lung may be extremely important.

DRUGS

Sometimes the physician will want to give various cardiac drugs, usually when the back pressure down the pulmonary artery and into the right heart has produced actual right heart failure. Diuretics are often used to drain the excess fluid from the tissues through the kidneys. In some cases digitalis is very helpful, while in others it is not. Some drugs are claimed to be respiratory stimulants. In other words, it was hoped that they would actually stimulate the patient's depth and rate of breathing. These drugs have not been very successful and are not in wide use.

EXERCISE

Breathing is a muscular activity that is carried on mostly by the diaphragm, but it is aided by the muscles of the chest wall and of the shoulder girdle. By increasing the efficiency of these muscles the physician may make available to the patient the small amount of extra oxygen that can make the difference between health and invalidism.

These exercises cannot be described here in detail; however, they can be useful but must be kept up for a long time under expert supervision. Exercise does not really change the basic lung disease in COPD or, indeed, in any form of chronic lung disease; what exercise can do, however, through the "conditioning" effect is to increase the efficiency of the delivery of blood to and through the lungs and hence increase the efficiency of oxygen uptake from the air. This increased efficiency lasts only as long as exercise is continued; a few weeks after exercise has been stopped, lung function returns to its previous state. The improved oxygen uptake with exercise, however, is sometimes so dramatic that it permits the patient to resume employment, go back to forms of recreation such as golf, walking, and the like, and begin leading a much more normal existence, and in these terms it is very well worthwhile. Whenever possible a supervised exercise program should be part of the rehabilitation of chronic lung disease.

Chronic cor pulmonale, then, is a form of heart disease that in the future may be largely eradicated by preventing or diminishing the various kinds of lung disease that produce it. This means treating infections in the lungs promptly, controlling asthma, avoiding exposure to various toxins, and, above all, *stopping cigarette smoking.*

Even when chronic cor pulmonale has progressed to significant or dangerous stages, modern therapy can still offer considerable relief of symptoms and can sometimes provide the patient years of comfortable, useful, active life.

13 Infectious heart disease

Infection and inflammation may attack the heart just as they may attack any of the other tissues of the body. The bacteria that cause pneumonia, boils, wound infections, appendicitis, sinusitis, meningitis, or any of their kindred infections can also attack the heart. The viruses of influenza, infectious mononucleosis (glandular fever), poliomyelitis, measles, chickenpox, or any of a hundred familiar virus infections also can attack the heart in any of its layers. At this point the word "layers" should be defined (Chapter 1). If you cut open the chest and looked at the heart you would see first of all a sack of tissue, very much like a heavy plastic bag, which surrounds the heart just as a clear, heavy plastic grocery bag might hold a cantaloupe. This sack of tissue, called the **pericardium,** forms a loose protective layer around the heart. When the pericardium is infected or inflamed, the disease is called **pericarditis.** If you cut open the pericardial sac, you see the main mass of the heart muscle itself, the **myocardium.** Infection or inflammation here is called **myocarditis.** Cutting the heart itself open, you find the lining of the heart covered with a shiny, slick, wet membrane, much like the lining of the mouth. This is called the **endocardium,** and infection here is called **endocarditis.**

Some acute inflammations like rheumatic fever involve all three of these heart layers. The patient will have pericarditis, myocarditis, and endocarditis all at once. This is a special case and it is best described in the chapter on rheumatic fever. It is more common to find inflammation of each heart layer as a separate disease with its own distinct character and significance (Figs. 13-1 and 13-2). These inflammations will be described separately for that reason.

PERICARDITIS

Imagine that the influenza virus attacks the lining of the pericardium. Picture the lining of the pericardium as something looking much like the back of a person's throat. When the virus attacks this membrane, it will look similar to a severe sore throat. The tissue first becomes red and swollen and pus or mucus may form in large quantities. Sometimes clear fluid may form, much like the clear fluid that runs out of one's nose during a severe cold. There is a difference, of course. One cannot cough up this mucus or blow out this fluid into a handkerchief because it is trapped in a sac around the heart with nowhere to go. There will almost always be some kind of pain in the chest that will partly come and go with breathing. The amount of pain will depend on the amount of fluid or mucus in the sac around the heart. If a great deal of this material piles up, the heart is actually compressed so that it cannot pump very well, and the patient now becomes quite ill. In the mild cases the patient may feel as if he had an ordinary bout of the **flu,** with the difference that there will be some discomfort somewhere in the front of his chest.

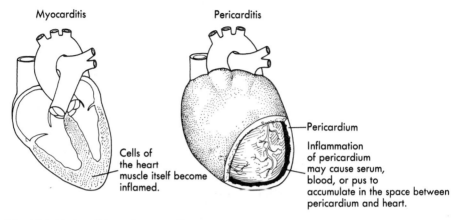

Fig. 13-1. Pericarditis and myocarditis. Inflammation of the sac around the heart, the pericardium, or of the heart muscle itself, the myocardium.

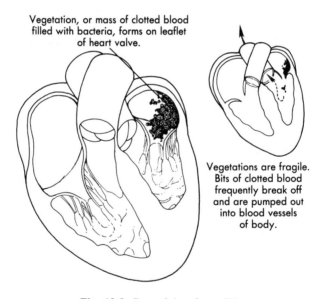

Fig. 13-2. Bacterial endocarditis.

Diagnosing pericarditis is usually easy if the physician can use the electrocardiogram and the fluoroscope in addition to physical examination. Sometimes the diagnosis can be made with a stethoscope alone. Often the physician will need to record electrocardiograms for three or four days in succession to decide that pericarditis is or is not present.

How serious is pericarditis? This depends almost entirely on the amount of material that piles up, or accumulates, in the sac around the heart and on the kind of material. The kind of material, in turn, depends on the kind of germ doing the infecting and on the patient's immune response to the germ. Sometimes pus forms in great quantities, and the patient's course will then be **septic,** with high fever and chilling; he may be in considerable danger from the infection itself. In other cases bloody fluid or clear, thin fluid may accumulate, and the chief problem is the compression of the heart when the large quantity of fluid has actually distended the pericardium. Treatment of this disease is based first on destruction of the infecting bacteria or germ when possible and second on the removal of the blood, pus, or fluid that as accumulated around the heart. This is often done by inserting a large needle through the chest wall and into the pericardial sac. The physician withdraws the fluid by means of a large syringe. In severe cases this may have to be done a number of times, and sometimes a small incision must be made in the chest wall for better drainage.

For most of the ordinary bacteria, such as the pneumonia germ, the staphylococcus, and the streptococcus, the physician can use antibiotics from sulfonamides through penicillin to the broad-spectrum antibiotics of various kinds. What is used will always depend on the kind of bacteria or germ present.

If the infection is caused by a virus, the problem is more difficult; there is nothing at this time known to science that will kill a virus in one's body. The patient's own natural immunity must do this in any virus disease. This is true in measles, chickenpox, influenza, encephalitis, or any of the familiar virus diseases; it is also true in viral infections of the pericardium. A virus is an extremely tiny form of life, much smaller than the ordinary "germ," or bacterium. Nothing is known as yet that can be given by injection or taken by pill that will destroy viruses inside the human body, but fortunately the patient's own body usually does the job. In viral pericarditis the physician will be concerned mostly about the amount of fluid in the pericardial sac. If it accumulates in dangerous quantities, it must be removed.

Rheumatic fever is one of an entire group of diseases called **collagen diseases.** These are diseases that affect the tissues that hold the body together, the fine connective tissues around the joints, between the muscles, and along the course of the blood vessels. Several mysterious diseases somehow related to rheumatic fever fall into this group. These include lupus erythematosus, polyarteritis nodosa, and several very rare related forms of illness. Most of the collagen diseases can also produce pericarditis. When they do, the physician will often use steroids such as cortisone to suppress the inflammation in the tissues. Rheumatic pericarditis is well described in Chapter 11 and needs no further mention here.

When some kinds of pericarditis heal, they leave a great deal of scar tissue behind, which "glues" the pericardium tightly around the heart. The pericardial membrane is actually bound down to the heart by masses of scar tissue that form broad adhesions. When this happens, the patient may go into heart failure because the heart simply cannot beat very well. Imagine putting your hand into a boxing glove that had been thoroughly stiffened with glue. Imagine then trying to open and shut your fist in such a way as to squeeze a bulb syringe. Obviously you could squeeze a little, but you couldn't squeeze very much or very efficiently. This is what happens when the pericardium is bound down around the heart in the condition called **adhesive,** or **constrictive, pericarditis.** It is always the result of some type of acute pericarditis. The outcome here is happy, since it is now possible to operate on the patient, cut away the scar tissue, and leave him a normal heart that functions as well as it did before he became ill.

There are no particular ways of preventing pericarditis; it simply appears out of the blue. When tuberculosis was common not so many years ago, tuberculous pericarditis was the most feared form of this disease. Tuberculous pericarditis was once so common that physicians were told to regard all pericarditis as tuberculous until proved otherwise. Control of tuberculosis in the last two decades has made tuberculous pericarditis very rare. This is a happy phenomenon because it was a very dangerous disease. Most of the cases of pericarditis the physician sees today are caused by viruses, by collagen disease of some kind, or by no cause that can be found at all. In the great majority of cases the disease is not particularly severe, and the patient makes a complete recovery.

MYOCARDITIS

The term "myocarditis" has a curious medical history. Physicians have known for a long time that such diseases as rheumatic fever or diptheria caused inflammation of the heart muscle, properly called myocarditis. Unfortunately the medical profession had a tendency to call a lot of other diseases myocarditis some thirty or forty years ago for lack of a better name or for lack of accurate diagnosis. A great deal of coronary artery disease, for example, was lumped into the wastebasket, and the term "myocarditis" fell into bad repute. It is a perfectly proper term when used correctly, and it certainly is a common disease.

Any of the viruses or bacteria described so far can also attack the cells of the heart muscle. The heart muscle can also become inflamed in the course of any of the collagen diseases. Diagnosing myocarditis is difficult and sometimes impossible. The seriousness of the disease varies. It may be a very slight inflammation of the muscle cells that produces only a sense of fatigue and of rapid pounding of the heart, while at the other end of the scale it may be a fatal illness. Careful studies recently have shown that many of the common respiratory viruses that produce fever, aches, cough, and "scratchy throats," usually miscalled "flu," can and do attack the heart muscle, producing myocarditis. A large porportion of patients with poliomyelitis, when this disease was prevalent, probably had some degree of myocarditis.

As in the case of pericarditis you must picture the heart muscle looking much like a sore throat, with red, inflamed, swollen tissues. If inflammation of the muscle cells becomes severe, their pumping efficiency drops; the patient may go into congestive heart failure. Some types of myocarditis heal completely, leaving the heart muscle about as good as new, while others leave pernament scarring behind, which weakens the action of the heart.

Again, there isn't much the patient can do to prevent myocarditis of the common types. This is not true of rheumatic myocarditis, since rheumatic fever is at least partly preventable. Chapter 11 covers this adequately. If a patient finds that his recovery from a case of flu is unusually slow, if the same patient notices that it is hard to breathe when he walks along the street, or if he notices further that his heart seems to pound quite a long time after walking up a few stairs, the patient is at least a possible candidate for some kind of myocarditis. He should consult his physician, who can check to see if there has been, in fact, any inflammation of the heart muscle. Remember this is a difficult diagnosis much of the time, and the patient may have to go through repeated electrocardiograms, x-ray examinations, and physical checks to see what is going on.

Treatment depends on the kind of bacteria, virus, or disease causing the myocarditis. It also depends on the severity of the inflammation. Antibiotics, steroids, digitalis, oxygen, and all the usual measures for combating congestive heart failure may have to come into play.

INFECTIOUS ENDOCARDITIS

Inflammation of the lining surface of the heart, the membrane that coats the ventricles and covers the valves, is very different. Much of it can be prevented, and many cases are now curable. This is quite a change. When I was in medical school, nobody had ever survived an infection of the endocardium, or endocarditis, in all medical history; in every case the victim died.

Endocarditis divides into two categories, the subacute, which means a long drawn-out, slow, smoldering disease, and the acute, which means an overwhelming, sudden infection. In each case the germs attack the endocardium covering the heart valves. They form tiny clusters on the valves that grow much like a fungus growing on the trunk of a tree. As the germs grow and multiply, blood clots form about them, providing further shelter and nourishment for the bacteria. These clots, teeming with bacteria, sometimes become as large as the end of one's finger. They are called **vegetations** because of their resemblance to a fungus or to some similar kind of plant life (Fig. 13-2).

These vegetations are exceedingly dangerous for several reasons; for one thing they are extremely soft with the consistency of a lump of gelatin, and hence are very fragile. Sooner or later the torrent of blood pouring through the heart will break bits of these vegetations off, and then there is a blood clot loaded with disease-causing bacteria floating out into the blood vessels of the body. Sometimes whole showers of these clots are pumped out at one time. The patient who has these clots floating through his arteries is sitting on a fused time bomb. First, if the clots are large, they will block an artery somewhere, causing death of the tissue that the artery supplies. This may happen in the brain, the spleen, the kidneys, the hands, the legs, the bowel, or any part of the body to which the blood flows. Second, each of these clots is a floating mass of infection. Bacteria swarm within it, ready to start an abscess wherever they lodge.

The patient suffering from the subacute form of endocarditis will usually notice low-grade fever, which may come and go for days or weeks. Finally, clots will lodge somewhere, often producing drastic symptoms that make the diagnosis painfully obvious. These clots may be so small that they produce only tiny discolored blotches under the nails or in the skin. The physician who knows the patient has a heart murmur and who finds that patient running a low-grade fever will instantly become suspicious of endocarditis and will start testing the blood for infecting bacteria. Determination that vegetations are present can also be made by the difference these growths make in the heart sounds. A heart murmur will usually be heard, and the character of this murmur will tend to change from day to day as the vegetation grows or changes shape.

Before the discovery of penicillin nobody ever recovered from this type of endocarditis. Bit by bit the patient was hammered to death by septic blood clots that lodged in the vital organs of the body until the patient died. Sometimes the patient died of heart failure from the tremendous growth of vegetations within the heart before any blood clots could travel to the vital organs. The acute form of endocarditis is very similar to the subacute except that it happens more swiftly, with sudden, devastating effects. The vegetations grow quickly, the fever is very high; in the days before antibiotics the patient was critically ill and usually died within a few days.

In most patients subacute or "long, drawn-out" endocarditis can now be prevented or, if not, often can be cured. Many of these infections take place in people whose heart valves bear the scars of rheumatic fever. Certain congenital heart abnormalities also predispose to this disease: so does the various forms of degeneration that attack the heart valves in older patients.

In recent years a great many cases of acute infectious endocarditis were the result of injection of infected material into the veins by narcotic addicts. In a large study in a general hospital (Los Angeles County, University of Southern California Medical Center) the incidence of infectious endocarditis was 1 out of 1,609 cases. Thirty-five cases in this one-year period occurred in young addicts, while twenty-eight cases occurred in patients with established heart disease. Of the thirty-five addicts, seven (20%) died.

Patients who have an artifical heart valve in place must guard with great care against infectious endocarditis, since infecting organisms are very likely to lodge on the plastic and metal components of the artificial valve.

Most cases of subacute bacterial endocarditis are caused by a common germ found in almost everyone's mouth. This germ usually invades the bloodstream after some dental operation. In recent years other types of organisms have been detected as causes of endocarditis in increasing numbers. Many of these are "gram-negative" (appear pink when stain for microsopic examination by the Gram method) organisms, which are much more difficult to treat than the streptococcus.

How can one prevent this frightfully dangerous disease? Some remarkably simple logical preventive measures will give almost 100% protection.

1. Patients known to have diseased valves or who have an artificial valve in place should receive large doses of penicillin before, during, and after any dental procedure on any area of the mouth that may even by slightly infected. (This probably applies even to the cleaning of teeth.) If the patient is allergic to penicillin, other antibiotics can be used.

2. Patients with diseased valves who are to undergo any invasive procedure in an area potentially contaminated must receive antibiotic prophylaxis with agents suitable for the bacteria that may be encountered. Examination of the bladder with a cystoscope, examination of the

bowel with a sigmoidoscope or colonoscope, or possibly examination of an infected lung with a bronchoscope all represent invasions of potentially infected areas that may release bacteria into the bloodstream. The physician performing the procedure will have a reasonable idea of the kind of bacteria that may be encountered and can prescribe appropriate antibiotics. However, the patient who knows that a diseased heart valve is present would always do well to remind the physician, since this detail can get overlooked in the stress of heavy scheduling.

3. Pregnant women with known valvular disease should receive the same preventive antibiotic treatment before, during, and after delivery. The risk of endocarditis during and after delivery is very great if preventive measures are not taken.

4. Narcotic addicts should attain some minimal degree of realization of the awful danger to which they expose themselves when they inject infected material into their bloodstream. It should be possible for even the most hardened addict to understand that death is quite likely to follow.

These precautions apply to all forms of congenital heart disease except for the simple secundum type of atrial septal defect. (See Chapter 16, Congenital Heart Disease.)

Dental infections are not the only way that these bacteria may enter the bloodstream, but they are the principal and most common ones. By slamming the door on this one avenue of infection, one probably prevents three fourths of all cases of subacute bacterial endocarditis.

Acute endocarditis is caused by a different set of bacteria. The most common organism here is the familiar staphylococcus, the same bacterium that is often found in boils and abscesses. Proper administration of the right antibiotic in the presence of known infection becomes ten times more important in people known to have disease of the heart valves. Older people with chalky or calcific disease of the heart valves often suffer endocarditis of either type.

Treatment in the past was surprisingly successful. During the 1940s and 1950s there was a very significant decrease in the mortality rate (to about 20%) thanks to the use of potent antibiotics on a group of bacteria that was easily destroyed.

In the past decade the mortality rate has again increased largely because of increased infection with resistant bacteria and the very high incidence of infection caused by drug addiction. (Most tragically this last group consists chiefly of young people.)

When a physician treats endocarditis, the bacteria that caused the infection must be grown artificially so that they can be identified. These bacteria must then be tested against various antibiotics to see which will kill them and what amount will be needed; only then can the physician proceed intelligently to destroy the infection. Treatment may be a long, drawn-out process because huge doses of penicillin or other antibiotics are often needed over long periods of time —rarely less than six weeks. After the initial successes of the 1940s and 1950s it must be repeated that the disease is again becoming more dangerous. It is still heartening to realize that a disease that had killed every one of its victims in the history of humanity until the discovery of penicillin has now been at least in part conquered. The temporary setback of the 1960s and 1970s has been sociologic and not a medical one.

Remember the important message of this section: anybody who has had valvular disease of any kind should always receive adequate doses of appropriate antibiotics before surgery or instrumentation in any potentially infected area of the body. The same is true of women facing childbirth. Most types of congenital deformity of the heart also require endocarditis prophylaxis.

Always inform your dentist and physician of the fact that you have structural abnormality of the heart before any dental, surgical or obstetric procedure is undertaken.

14 Heart block and the sick sinus: pacemakers

The electrobiologic system that generates the electric force of the heartbeat and conducts that force through the tissues of the heart is formed of living cells; like all other tissues in the body these cells will inevitably grow old; they may be attacked by any of a number of diseases, and they may die altogether. As a result the heart may beat very slowly or may stop beating altogether. This will happen basically for one of two reasons:

1. "Generator" failure: failure of the sinus node to generate the activating impulse of the heart adequately—the "sick sinus" syndrome.
2. Conductor failure: failure of the conducting tissues to transmit the activating electric impulse from one part of the heart to another; this usually means failure of transmission from atria to ventricles—heart block.

THE SICK SINUS SYNDROME

Remember that the sinoatrial node functions like the coil in a car, generating the electric force that begins the heart cycle. The cells in the sinoatrial node that actually produce this electric potential may degenerate and fail to fire often enough for the needs of the heart. More commonly, a tiny area of block may form within the sinoatrial node; certain cells that are supposed to conduct this impulse out to the atria and start it on its way may undergo degenerative changes so that they function only slowly or erratically. Thus the electric potential dies at birth; it never breaks out into the atria. This kind of failure is called "exit block" because the impulse never gets the chance to "exit" into the conducting tissues of the atria and thence across the heart.

When this happens the sinoatrial node is described simply as "sick," and the syndrome is called the "sick sinus syndrome." Subnormal sinus node function may take several forms:

1. Sinoatrial exit block. An occasional electric impulse will fail to break out of the sinus node into the atria, and there will be a pause in the heartbeat that will be exactly twice as long as the normal interval between beats. The reason for this is that the pacemaker cells go on firing whether their impulse is conducted out to the atria or not, and so the next impulse that is conducted will be right on schedule. The length of the pause may be double the normal rate, triple, or even longer, but it will be some exact multiple of the basic heart rate. This is called **sinoatrial exit block.**

Sometimes sinoatrial exit block takes complicated forms with variable lengths of pauses because of varying degrees of exit block within the tiny structure. Only a cardiologist with particular skill in the field of cardiac arrhythmias can really analyze some of these tracings.

2. Erratic sinus pauses. Sometimes the sinus node may pause in an unpre-

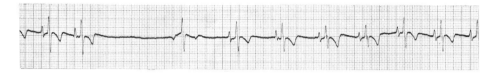

Fig. 14-1. Sinoatrial exit block. The second P wave is followed by an abrupt pause, lasting about 3 seconds, ended by an ectopic beat. Then the sinus rhythm resumes. Many pauses of this type accompanying symptoms might suggest "sick sinus" syndrome but would not prove the diagnosis per se.

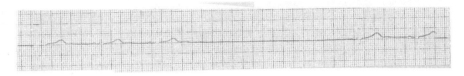

Fig. 14-2. Sinus pause. There is an abrupt pause in the sinus rhythm lasting for almost 15 seconds.

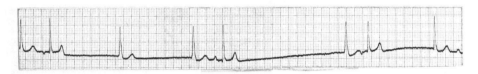

Fig. 14-3. Extreme sinus bradycardia. There is only one normal sinus beat on the whole strip. All the other beats arise from an ectopic focus in the region of the AV node.

dictable manner for long periods—that is, several seconds or more. These erratic pauses that are not multiples of the basic rate may be the result of failure of the pacemaker cells themselves rather than of the conducting tissues.

3. Persistent bradycardia. The word "bradycardia" simply means a slow heart rate; by convention any rate below 60 is called a bradycardia. If the heart rate remains abnormally slow at all times and if the heart is not able to respond with a normal rate increase to such demands as exertion, it is good evidence that the sinoatrial node is "sick": that is, discharging at an inappropriately slow rate for the needs of the body (Figs. 14-1 to 14-3).

Symptoms of "bradycardia" or "slow heart rate" type of sick sinus syndrome

When the heart beats too slowly for the needs of the body or when it pauses for an abnormally long time, there may be failure of delivery of blood to the tissues of the brain and the patient will notice symptoms of dizziness (vertigo) or of actual fainting (syncope).

Vertigo or syncope may come on quite unpredictably during a sinus pause or during a period of sinoatrial exit block; if the patient suffers from sustained

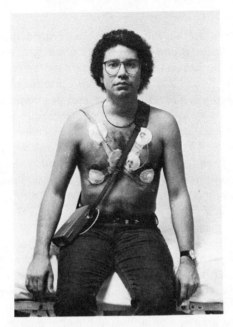

Fig. 14-4. Patient wearing Holter monitor recording equipment.

sinus bradycardıa, the syncope or vertigo may be noted during work or exercise, times when the heart would normally be expected to increase its rate. Because of the inadequate sinus node function, the heart cannot increase its rate enough for the extra demand, and the patient may notice symptoms of inadequate blood flow to the brain, again, vertigo or syncope.

The patient may suspect a sick sinus syndrome *when there are symptoms of sudden dizziness or actual fainting.* These symptoms may come on at random for no obvious reason or may be brought on consistently by some form of physical exertion.

Diagnosis of the bradycardia or "slow heartbeat" type of sick sinus syndrome can be made only when the electrocardiogram records one of the types of abnormally slow heartbeat described here *at the time the patient actually feels symptoms.* This can be done by recording long strips of a conventional electrocardiogram, by observing an oscilloscope in a monitored bed in an intensive or coronary care unit, or by having the patient wear a machine called a Holter monitor, which records the electrocardiogram continuously for 12 or 24 hours (Fig. 14-4). The patient simply wears this machine slung over one shoulder, much as one would wear a binoculars or camera case, while recording electrodes are pasted to the chest. If symptoms appear, the patient jots down the time and character of these symptoms in a diary, and the physician later "plays back" the electrocardiogram with the aid of a computer so that he can scan the entire 24 hours of electrocardiographic recording and correlate the symptoms with the changes, if any, in heart rhythm at that time.

CAVEATS

• *It must be proved that the pauses in heart rate actually are producing the symptoms because dizziness and fainting very often have nothing to do with the heart and would not be helped at all by insertion of the pacemaker.*

• *How slow is "slow"? It is not at all unusual for the pulse rate to drop to low levels during sleep when the body's demands are minimal; a pulse rate in the 40s is quite common in the average 24-hour electrocardiographic recording. Well-trained athletes with excellent cardiac performance will also have very slow pulse rates simply because they have very efficient hearts that do not have to beat many times per minute to produce a normal cardiac output.*

• *Pauses in sinus node discharge are not at all rare and become significant only if they are actually correlated with the production of symptoms.*

Risk

The bradycardia type of sick sinus syndrome is not really a risk to life per se. The danger comes if a patient loses consciousness while driving a car, crossing a busy street, or performing some hazardous occupation such as working at a height or around dangerous moving machinery. In older patients particularly there is always the danger of a fall with a resulting broken bone such as a hip, which can produce a long and complicated hospital course.

Treatment

The only treatment of a proved symptomatic "bradycardia" type of sick sinus syndrome is the insertion of a pacemaker to the heart. There is no form of medical therapy known that can cause the sinus node to improve its function to any significant degree.

The slow-fast type of sick sinus syndrome

A sick sinus syndrome may appear in another form; in addition to the abnormally slow discharge of the sinus node there may be periods of very rapid heartbeat. This rapid beating will be caused by one of the three types of fast, abnormal atrial rhythms—either atrial fibrillation, atrial flutter, or paroxysmal atrial tachycardia (Chapter 5).

The periods of rapid beating will usually be brief—a few seconds or possibly minutes—especially early in the course of the disease. The patient will often feel an uncomfortable pounding sensation in the chest or have the feeling that the heart "is running away with itself." If the patient has coronary artery disease or if left ventricular function is subnormal, the periods of rapid beating may be accompanied by anginal pain or shortness of breath (Fig. 14-5).

When the rapid beating stops, the abnormally slow sinus rhythm will again appear, with single pauses or with a continuous slow rhythm.

The medical term for a rate below 60 is "bradycardia"; a rate above 100 is called "tachycardia"; the official medical name for this syndrome, therefore, is bradycardia-tachycardia form of sick sinus syndrome.

Nobody knows exactly why these periods of rapid beating are seen in association with subnormal sinus node function. It certainly isn't simply the slow

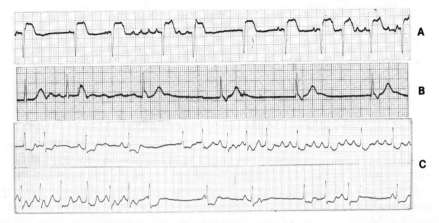

Fig. 14-5. The bradycardia-tachycardia form of sick sinus syndrome. **A,** Atrial fibrillation. **B,** Atrial flutter. **C,** Paroxysmal supraventricular tachycardia.

rate, since many healthy individuals have slow heart rates all their lives without any other abnormality of rhythm. The answer is probably that the degeneration that has depressed the function of the sinus node has also involved the other conducting systems in the atria. The normal electric controls are lost and the electrically unstable, diseased tissues will erupt with great periods of rapid rhythm.

Treatment for the "brady-tachy" syndrome is more complicated than for the simple "bradycardia" form of sick sinus.

1. A ventricular pacemaker is inserted to control the periods of slow rhythm.
2. Intensive drug management is used to control the rapid atrial rhythms.
3. When paroxysms of atrial flutter or fibrillation form the "tachy" part of the syndrome, the physician may want to consider long-term anticoagulant therapy because there is considerable danger of blood clots forming in the atria as they go in and out of the abnormal rhythm. When a blood clot grows in the atria, of course, a part of it may break off and be discharged out into the blood vessels of the body, with results that may well be catastrophic. For this reason if the atrial arrhythmia cannot be controlled with drugs, the physician may want to prescribe anticoagulants as long as the syndrome persists.

In the management of the tachy-brady syndrome it is usually necessary to record many electrocardiographic tracings or Holter monitor recordings to make sure that the rapid rhythm is, in fact, under control. In most cases the physician will have to do a great deal of adjusting drugs and doses before the rapid rhythms can be brought completely under control.

Pacemaker insertion for the sick sinus syndrome: questions and cautions

Insertion of a pacemaker in the heart to generate an artificial beat is the only satisfactory way to treat the slow, or bradycardia, type of sick sinus syndrome; before pacemakers were invented, no real treatment was available.

Unfortunately this boon to medical science is being abused; the sick sinus syndrome is being overdiagnosed and pacemakers are being overutilized. The physician who was the first to discover this syndrome and recognize its significance (Dr. Bernard Lown of Harvard University) has commented that at a rough guess about 80% of the pacemakers being inserted for supposed sick sinus syndrome are unnecessary. *In the United States today the sick sinus syndrome is the commonest diagnosis cited as justification for insertion of a permanent pacemaker. Careful reviews of current performance indicate that the sick sinus syndrome is being "overdiagnosed"—in other words, physicians are diagnosing sick sinus syndrome when it does not actually exist or when it is so mild that it is not significant and does not require pacemaker insertion. In many areas physicians appear to be diagnosing sick sinus syndrome when, in fact, the patient is simply showing the effect of one of several cardiac drugs such as propranolol or digitalis which almost always depress sinus node function to some extent. The diagnosis of sick sinus syndrome should never be attempted while the patient is taking a drug that depresses sinus node function.* In a large eastern medical center physicians recently instituted very strict review of every case alleged to need a pacemaker; by simply insisting on the criteria outlined on pp. 176 to 179 before pacemaker insertion was permitted, the review committee reduced the number of implantations by 70% within two years. Other review groups have had much the same experience.

However, consider the other face of the coin: a true sick sinus syndrome can be distressing and even disabling. Accurate diagnosis and adequate treatment (by pacing) can produce some of the most remarkable beneficial results in terms of life and function in all modern cardiology.

Be sure the diagnosis is thoroughly substantiated then don't hesitate to go ahead with treatment.

ATRIOVENTRICULAR BLOCK

The heart may beat slowly or stop altogether because of failure of conduction of the electric impulse from the atria to the ventricles. This is what most physicians mean when they speak of "heart block." *After years of speaking about this subject to medical audiences all across the United States I am convinced that a substantial number of physicians do not really understand atrioventricular block well enough to make specific recommendations to their patients. They often do not understand exactly where the block is in the atrioventricular conducting system or what it means in terms of risk and treatment. This section of the book will try to do something that has never been done before: it will attempt to explain to the patient without any medical training exactly what the types of atrioventricular block are, the risks associated with each type, and the appropriate forms of treatment. This may seem alarmingly technical, but don't worry: any intelligent reader should be able to grasp the subject sufficiently for all practical purposes in an hour or two of careful study.*

Typical electrocardiographic tracings of the various kinds of blocks are in-

cluded here; in many cases by simply counting the number of little squares between one wave and another you will be able to decide what kind of heart block is present and where it is in the atrioventricular conducting system. For the patient contemplating pacemaker insertion, this may be a couple of hours well spent.

Anatomy of the atrioventricular conducting system (Fig. 14-6)

The atrioventricular conducting system begins with a single "strand" or mass of conducting cells connecting the bottom of the atria with the top of the ventricles. Because it connects atria with ventricles, it is logically called the atrioventricular node or as is usually abbreviated, the AV node.

Through most of its course the AV node is a complex mass of intertwining cells; under a very high-power microscope it looks like a dense spider web. At the bottom of the node the cells start to "straighten out" and run in little parallel tubules, or canals. This bottom part of the AV node was first described by two investigators named His and Tarawa; it is commonly referred to as the **bundle of His.**

The bundle of His divides into two branches, one running down each side of the intraventricular septum. These are called the **bundle branches,** left and right. The left bundle branch carries the electric impulse to the left ventricle, the right bundle to the right. As the bundle branches course out through the ventricles they divide into smaller and smaller twigs, ending finally in tiny structures called Purkinje fibers.

The atrioventricular conducting system thus has three simple elements—the single strand formed by the AV node and its bottom portion, the His bundle, and the two bundle branches. The left bundle branch appears to have two divisions, or fascicles (the word "fascicle" comes from the Latin word "fasces," meaning rods or sticks); one conducts the electric impulse forward and to the right across the left ventricle and the other backward and to the left.

It is very important to remember that the two bundle branches are separate structures, each with its own individual blood supply. They are no more connected to each other than the left arm is to the right arm. Abnormality of one bundle branch does not imply abnormality of the other any more than a cut on the left arm would imply a cut on the right.

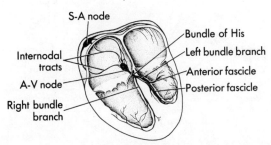

Fig. 14-6. Anatomy of the atrioventricular conducting system.

Speed of conduction

Conduction through the AV node is very slow; in the adult heart the interval from the beginning of atrial activation (the beginning of the P wave) and the end of passage through the AV node (the first spike of the ventricular complex) will never be less than 0.12 second, or three small squares on the electrocardiogram. This interval is called the P-R (atria-to-ventricles) interval: normal passage time is somewhere between 0.12 second (three squares) and 0.20 second (five squares) (Fig. 14-7).

How to measure time on an electrocardiogram

Each small square on the paper represents 0.04 seconds.
Each large square includes five small ones; therefore
each large square equals
5 × 0.04 or 0.20 second.

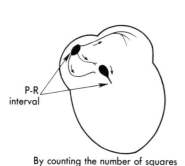

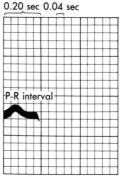

P-R interval

By counting the number of squares from the beginning of the P wave to the ventricular complex the cardiologist can determine the time it takes the activating wave to move across the atria and through the A-V node to the beginning of the bundle branch system.

The P-R interval is normally 0.20 or less.

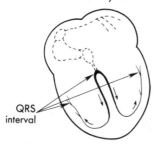

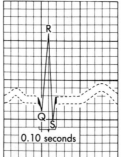

QRS interval

The width of the ventricular complex tells how long it takes the activating wave to move throughout the entire ventricular activating network.

The QRS or ventricular complex is normally 0.10 or less wide.

Fig. 14-7. Normal electrocardiographic time intervals.

Conduction in the bundle-branch system is very rapid—about four meters per second; this is the reason the electric complex inscribed during ventricular activation is narrow. (The width of the QRS, or ventricular activating complex, represents the time it takes the electric impulse to travel all the way through the ventricular conducting system from the beginning of the bundle branches to the end of the Purkinje fibers. This is normally about 0.08 to 0.10 second, or 2 to 2½ small squares on the electrocardiogram.)

Note that by simply counting the small squares, each of which equals 0.04 seconds, it is possible to measure the time it takes an impulse to travel from the sinus node all the way through the AV node (the PR interval) and from the beginning of the bundle-branch system to the end of the ventricular conducting system (the width of the QRS, or ventricular activating complex).

Delay or failure of conduction from atria to ventricles can therefore take place in the single strand of tissue that constitutes the AV node-His bundle combination or in the bundle-branch system (Fig. 14-8). It is important to remember that the bundle-branch system has *two* strands; if only one were diseased, the other bundle branch could conduct the electric impulse to the ventricles perfectly well. *Only if conduction through both bundle branches is interrupted will there be failure of conduction from atria to ventricles.*

Classes of atrioventricular block

Atrioventricular block will fall into one of three general classes that are quite sensible and easy to remember:

1. First-degree AV block. This means that every impulse starting in the sinus node reaches the ventricles and produces a response. It simply takes longer than normal getting there. The PR interval represents the time it takes an impulse to travel across the atria and down through the AV node to the ventricles; in first-

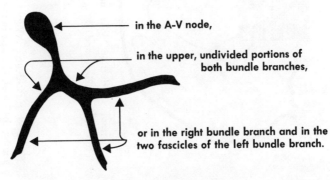

Delayed conduction or failure of conduction
from atria to ventricles may be the result of
disease or dysfunction in one of three sites:

in the A-V node,

in the upper, undivided portions of
both bundle branches,

or in the right bundle branch and in the
two fascicles of the left bundle branch.

Fig. 14-8. Places where atrioventricular block can occur.

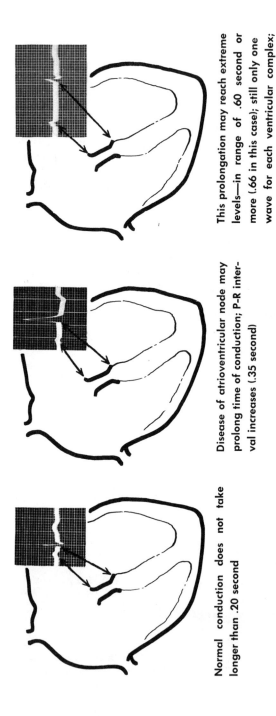

Normal conduction does not take longer than .20 second

Disease of atrioventricular node may prolong time of conduction; P-R interval increases (.35 second)

This prolongation may reach extreme levels—in range of .60 second or more (.66 in this case); still only one wave for each ventricular complex; P-R interval constant

Fig. 14-9. First-degree AV block. The normal narrow QRS complex shows that the bundle-branch system is functioning normally; the block must be in the AV node–His bundle region.

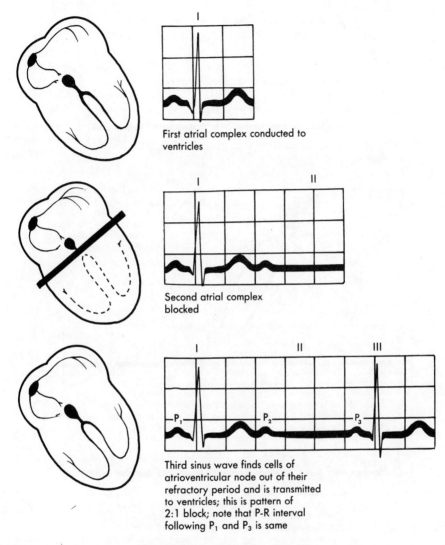

First atrial complex conducted to ventricles

Second atrial complex blocked

Third sinus wave finds cells of atrioventricular node out of their refractory period and is transmitted to ventricles; this is pattern of 2:1 block; note that P-R interval following P_1 and P_3 is same

Fig. 14-10. Second-degree block.

degree AV block the PR interval is prolonged (Fig. 14-9). Since the upper limit of normal for conduction from atria to ventricles is 0.20 second, or five squares, a PR interval of six, seven, or eight squares (0.24 to 0.32 second) is clearly abnormal and means that the electric impulse is taking too long moving from atria to ventricles (Fig. 14-10).

   2. Second-degree AV block. Some atrial impulses reach the ventricles and produce a response and some do not. The ones which do not are blocked in some part of the atrioventricular conducting system. This will happen because the cells in some part of this system are diseased and cannot conduct as many times per

Complete atrioventricular block in the A-V node.

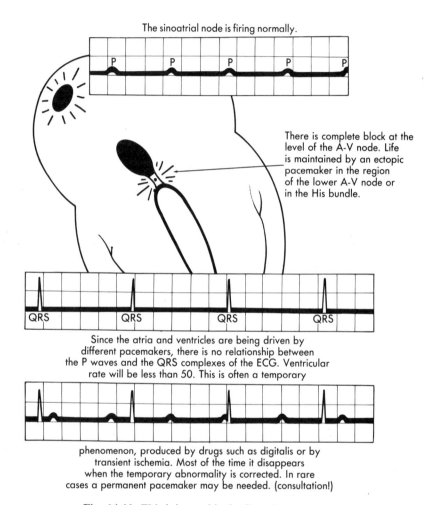

The sinoatrial node is firing normally.

P   P   P   P   P

There is complete block at the
level of the A-V node. Life
is maintained by an ectopic
pacemaker in the region
of the lower A-V node or
in the His bundle.

QRS   QRS   QRS   QRS

Since the atria and ventricles are being driven by
different pacemakers, there is no relationship between
the P waves and the QRS complexes of the ECG. Ventricular
rate will be less than 50. This is often a temporary

phenomenon, produced by drugs such as digitalis or by
transient ischemia. Most of the time it disappears
when the temporary abnormality is corrected. In rare
cases a permanent pacemaker may be needed. (consultation!)

Fig. 14-11. Third-degree block. Complete heart block.

minute as normal cells can; the diseased cells require longer "rest periods" than
healthy ones and hence will conduct fewer impulses.

3. Third-degree AV block (Fig. 14-11). *No* impulses from the atria reach
the ventricles. Life is maintained only because one of the "reserve" pacemakers
of the heart somewhere below the site of the block begins firing and stimulates the
heart to a steady beat. These reserve pacemakers are actually the "ectopic" beats
referred to in Chapter 5 on cardiac arrhythmias; when there is complete heart
block these ectopic, or extra, pacemakers come into play as a lifesaving device.

First-degree block

Now solve some puzzles. Try to analyze the tracing in Fig. 14-12. The PR interval is prolonged (eight squares, or 0.32 second). There is therefore block be tween the atria and the ventricles. Each P wave is followed by a ventricular com plex at the same regular interval, but the interval is too long. The diagnosis is *first-degree block.*

Where's the block? The ventricular complex is narrow (0.09 second), meaning that the bundle branches are conducting *normally.* Conduction in the bundle-branch system is evaluated simply by looking at the width of the ventricu lar complex. If this width is normal (less than 0.11 second, or about 2¾ little squares), both bundle branches must be functioning normally. *The only way the ventricles can be activated rapidly, producing a narrow QRS, is for both bundle branches to be conducting normally; that is, for each bundle branch to activate its respective ventricle rapidly and at the same speed as the opposite bundle branch so that everything happens simultaneously and quickly.*

The block in this tracing, therefore, must be above the "fork in the road" that starts the bundle-branch system. It must be in the AV node.

Second-degree AV block (Fig. 14-13)

Every other P wave in this tracing is blocked; it is not followed by a ven tricular complex. The alternative P waves are conducted through the ventricles with a normal PR interval and a normal narrow QRS complex.

Where is the block? The ventricular complexes that are produced are nar row, that is, normal, meaning that the bundle-branch system is functioning nor mally. *The block is therefore in the AV node.*

This kind of block cannot be in the bundle-branch system. To imagine it you would have to suppose that both bundle branches failed to conduct at the same identical hundredth of a second by sheer coincidence and then resumed con duction absolutely normally on the alternate beats—an impossibility. This would be about like imagining a simultaneous power failure in New York and Toronto by pure coincidence at the same hundredth of a second, both light systems turn ing on simultaneously, again at the same hundredth of a second, and with this process many times repeated.

The narrow QRS complex therefore tells the physician that both bundle branches are conducting normally; the block must be in the AV node.

Wenckebach AV block (Fig. 14-14). Wenckebach AV block is the com monest type of second-degree AV block; its long name is surprisingly easy to remember. A long time ago Dr. Wenckebach described this characteristic kind of conduction delay in the AV node. Imagine the cells in the AV node to be a line of workmen, all sick with flu. These workmen are supposed to be passing 30-pound bricks from one end of a line to the other, that is, from atria to ven tricles. When they are healthy they can do this very rapidly—up to 108 or more times a minute—but now they are sick and weak. They pass brick number one through normally, but they take a lot longer passing the next one and longer still passing the next, simply because they become progressively more fatigued. Final ly the workmen are lying about, exhausted, refusing to pass anything at all until

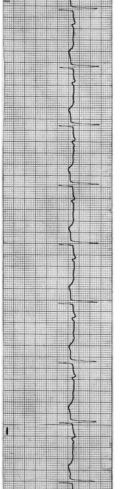

Fig. 14-12. First-degree block with narrow QRS. AV nodal block.

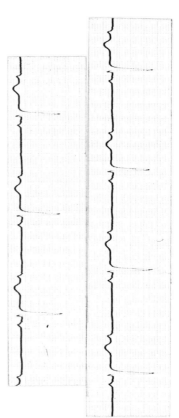

Fig. 14-13. Two-to-one block. The narrow QRS again tells the cardiologist that the bundle-branch system is firing normally and the block must be up in the AV node–His bundle region.

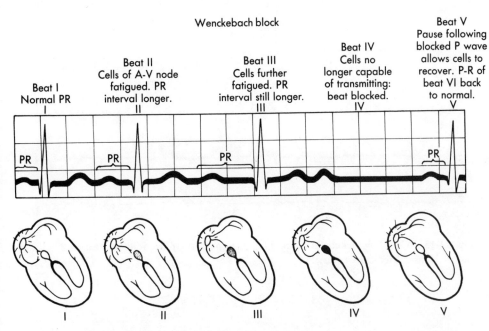

Fig. 14-14. Wenckebach AV block. Progressive fatigue of cells in the AV node until they fail to conduct entirely. The progressive fatigue before failure to conduct and the recovery of the cells during the pause after failure to conduct are characteristic of the Wenckebach phenomenon.

they've had a chance to rest. A brick arrives at the top of their line from the conveyor belt, but they ignore it. It doesn't get passed. It is blocked. After a rest the workmen have recovered and start passing their bricks along more rapidly, but the same cycle of progressive fatigue and final failure repeats itself.

This is a good picture of the Wenckebach type of atrioventricular block. The physician can tell that there is increasing fatigue of the cells in the AV node because the interval between the P wave and the ventricular response grows longer with each passage. Finally one P wave is not followed by a ventricular response; it is blocked. This failure of conduction through the AV node gives the cells a period of rest, and they resume conducting with a much shorter PR interval on the first beat after this period of rest.

Fig. 14-15 illustrates the Wenckebach phenomenon. The progressive prolongation of PR interval, meaning progressive fatigue of cells in the AV node, is obvious, as is the blocked P wave and the recovery after it.

Throughout, the QRS complex is narrow, meaning that the bundle-branch system is functioning normally; therefore the Wenckebach phenomenon must be taking place in the cells of the AV node.

Third-degree AV block, or complete AV block (Figs. 14-16 and 14-17)

The physician can diagnose complete AV block when there is no relationship at all between the P waves and the ventricular responses. The ectopic, or re-

90-year-old man receiving
digoxin, 0.25 mg/day

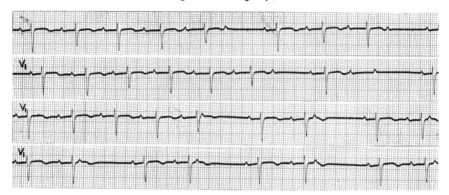

Fig. 14-15. ECG of Wenckebach block. (Tracing courtesy of Dr. William Nelson, University of Kansas Medical Center.)

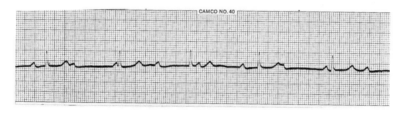

Fig. 14-16. Complete heart block in the AV node. The narrow ventricular complexes mean that the bundle-branch system is functioning normally.

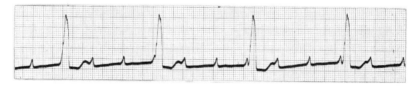

Fig. 14-17. Complete heart block in the bundle-branch system. Note wide ventricular complexes—the heart is being driven by an ectopic pacemaker in the ventricles.

serve, pacemaker driving the ventricles is discharging at its own natural rate, usually a good deal slower than the rate of the sinus node. Since none of the impulses from the sinus node are reaching the ventricles, the rate of the sinus node and the rate of the reserve pacemaker driving the ventricles are going to be completely different. There will be a completely helter-skelter relationship of P waves to ventricular responses (Fig. 14-11).

A trap for the unwary physician. One of the requirements for the diagnosis of complete AV block is a ventricular rate under 50. When the sinus node is firing somewhere in the normal range and the rate of the reserve, or ectopic, pace-

Atrioventricular dissociation without block
"pseudo-block"

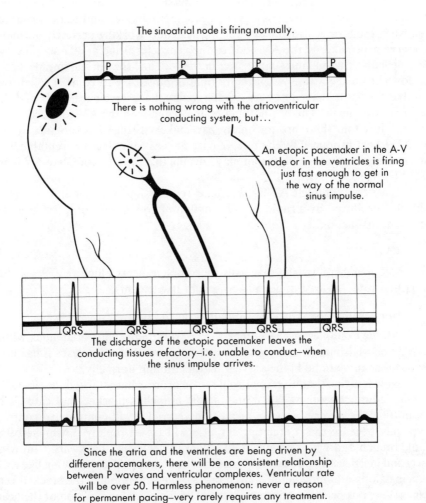

The sinoatrial node is firing normally.

There is nothing wrong with the atrioventricular
conducting system, but...

An ectopic pacemaker in the A-V
node or in the ventricles is firing
just fast enough to get in
the way of the normal
sinus impulse.

The discharge of the ectopic pacemaker leaves the
conducting tissues refractory—i.e. unable to conduct—when
the sinus impulse arrives.

Since the atria and the ventricles are being driven by
different pacemakers, there will be no consistent relationship
between P waves and ventricular complexes. Ventricular rate
will be over 50. Harmless phenomenon: never a reason
for permanent pacing—very rarely requires any treatment.

Fig. 14-18. Pseudo-complete block or interference association. This is a basically harmless rhythm when one of the reserve pacemakers of the heart begins firing rapidly enough to "get in the way of" the normal sinus impulse. The atria are driven by the normal sinus pacemaker and the ventricles are driven by an ectopic pacemaker. This should not be confused with true third-degree or complete heart block.

maker driving the ventricles is extremely slow, it is reasonable to suppose that there is plenty of time for an impulse to get through the AV conducting system between the beats of the reserve pacemaker and take over the rhythm. When it doesn't do so, the presumption is that there is block somewhere so that no impulses can reach the ventricles from the atria. If an ectopic pacemaker begins to drive the ventricles somewhere near the rate of the sinus node, a kind of "false block" may be produced. The ectopic pacemaker is not supposed to fire unless needed, but sometimes these tissues can become "irritable" and start discharging even when the atrioventricular conducting system is working perfectly normally. A reserve pacemaker in the AV node of the ventricles firing at 80 may take over the ventricular rhythm and simply "get in the way of" the normal impulses coming down from the atria. When the normal impulses try to come through they find that the tissues have just been discharged by the reserve pacemaker and they die an electric death. There is nothing really wrong with the AV conducting system; it's just that there are too many pacemakers firing. This doesn't do any harm; the beat produced by the reserve pacemaker is a perfectly acceptable beat, but the danger is that the physician may mistake this for true complete AV block (Fig. 14-18).

Since true complete AV block usually requires a pacemaker and the "pseudoblock" produced by a rapid ectopic rhythm almost never does, this is a very important distinction.

CAVEAT

• Remember that the diagnosis of complete heart block requires a slow ventricular rate—at least under 50—as one of its elements.

Block within the ventricles—bundle-branch block

All the examples of heart block shown so far have illustrated block within the AV node-His bundle complex. From the narrow QRS complexes it has been obvious that the bundle branch system is functioning normally.

Now imagine that disease or some toxic process has attacked the tissues of the bundle-branch system. When one bundle branch is blocked, not capable of transmitting the electric impulse at all, the ventricles will continue to contract adequately because the stimulating impulse will travel rapidly down the other bundle branch and will then invade the blocked ventricle "backward," moving slowly and inefficiently through the tissues of the blocked side, something like a car bouncing along a bumpy detour. Even though the activation of the blocked ventricle is slow, it is perfectly adequate in terms of the pumping function of the heart because the difference in time is only about four or five hundredths of a second.

The slow activation of the blocked ventricle is easy to detect on the electrocardiogram. Since the whole process of activating the ventricles is prolonged, the QRS, or ventricular complex, of the ECG will be wider than normal, reflecting this increase in activation time.

A great deal of experimental and clinical study has shown that when one bundle branch is blocked, the ventricular complex will always be 0.12 second

Bundle branch block

When only one bundle branch is blocked it isn't
very serious. The heart has a fail-safe system.

Conduction from atria to ventricles continues
through the other bundle branch, and rhythm
of the heart is not interrupted.

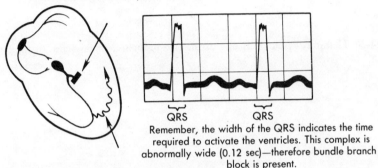

Remember, the width of the QRS indicates the time
required to activate the ventricles. This complex is
abnormally wide (0.12 sec)—therefore bundle branch
block is present.

The blocked ventricle is activated "backwards"
by a slow detour. This takes longer than normal
and the ventricular complex will therefore be
wider than usual (at least 0.12 seconds or 3 squares).

Fig. 14-19. Bundle-branch block.

wide, or equal to three small squares on the ECG. This is such a simple measurement that I like to tell medical students that if they can count to three, they can diagnose bundle-branch block. This is quite literally the case (Fig. 14-19).

Chronic block of one bundle branch is no great cause for immediate concern; many people live out a normal life span with a blocked bundle branch. However, if some kind of block now appears in the other bundle branch, the possibility of significant interruption of conduction from atria to ventricles becomes very real.

Hemiblocks, or fascicular blocks (Fig. 14-20)

Earlier it was noted that the left bundle branch is divided into two fascicles which conduct almost in opposite directions, rightward and leftward, front and back.

By looking at the electric direction of the electrocardiogram, the cardiologist can tell whether or not one of these fascicles is blocked. Considering conduction at the level of these fascicles, there are three strands of tissue connecting atria and ventricles; that is, the right bundle branch and the two divisions of the left. If, for example, the right bundle branch is blocked and one of the divisions of the left bundle branch is also blocked, there is now only half a bundle branch transmitting the exciting impulse from atria to ventricles. This kind of block is called bifascicular block. It is much commoner for the anterior rightward fascicle of the

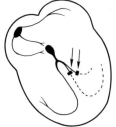

Either fascicle of the
left bundle branch may
be blocked—that is, it
may fail to conduct. The
heart will still be activated
through the remaining
conducting tissue and
the rhythm will not
be interrupted.

Fig. 14-20. Hemiblock; block of one of the two branches, or fascicles, of the left bundle branch.

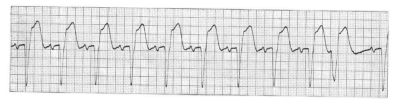

Fig. 14-21. Combination of bundle-branch block with first degree AV block.

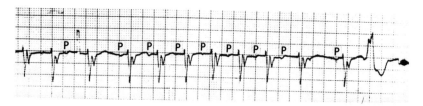

Fig. 14-22. Combination of bundle-branch block with Wenckebach block.

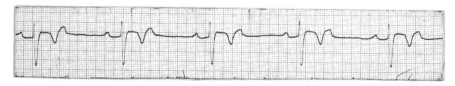

Fig. 14-23. Two-to-one "fixed ratio" block with bundle-branch block.

left bundle branch to suffer block than the posterior left one, which is a much stronger structure.

•   •   •

When one bundle branch is blocked, the appearance of any of the three types of atrioventricular block presents the cardiologist with two possibilities: (1) the delay in AV conduction may be within the AV node-His bundle strand, or (2) it may represent delayed conduction down the remaining bundle branch, since now there is no fail-safe double-conduction system in the ventricle. There is only one strand of conducting tissue connecting atria to ventricles and it consists of the AV node, the His bundle, and the one functioning bundle branch.

Is the atrioventricular block in the AV node-His bundle area, or is it a manifestation of disease in the remaining bundle branch? There are some clues in the electrocardiogram to help the cardiologist make this distinction.

First-degree AV block with bundle-branch block (Fig. 14-21)

The prolongation of the PR interval may represent delay in the AV node or in the other bundle branch. Looking at a tracing like Fig. 14-21, nobody could tell the difference.

Second-degree AV block

If the Wenckebach type of progressive AV block appears in a patient who already has one bundle branch blocked, the physician can be practically certain that the Wenckebach block is up in the AV node; it is extremely rare for the Wenchebach kind of progressive delay to appear in a bundle branch. The anatomic localization is almost 100% in the AV node (Fig. 14-22).

Two-to-one block

In Fig. 14-23 the P waves that do not reach the ventricles may be blocked in the atrioventricular node or in the other bundle branch. It is not possible to tell which from this tracing alone.

Mobitz type II block

Mobitz type II block (Fig. 14-24) is one of the most important kinds of block the physician has to recognize, and it is also the most widely misunderstood. When one bundle branch is blocked, the other bundle branch may suddenly fail from time to time, so that there is no conduction from atria to ventricles for one or more beats. *This failure will be abrupt; there will be no progressive fatigue before the blocked P wave and there will be no recovery afterward.* There is a kind of "all-or-none" conduction that is seen only in the bundle-branch system.

Therefore, when a cardiologist looks at the tracing of a patient with a preexisting bundle branch block and notices that occasional P waves are blocked *without any warning, without any preceding prolongation of the PR interval,* and with no recovery or shortening of the PR interval after the blocked wave, he can be quite certain that the failure to conduct from atria to ventricles is taking place in the one remaining bundle branch.

Mobitz II block

One bundle branch is permanently blocked.
Conduction from atria to the ventricles now depends
on one bundle branch. If the remaining bundle branch
fails, there will be no conduction from atria
to ventricles for
one or more beats.

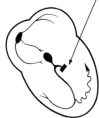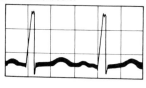

The distinction between Weckebach (A-V nodal) block and
Mobitz II (bundle branch) block is made with the ECG.

Mobitz II block

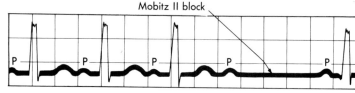

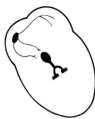

In Weckebach block there is always progressive
fatigue of the A-V node before it fails. There
is always "recovery" after the blocked P
wave. In Mobitz II block the failure
of conduction is abrupt. There is no warning
prolongation of P-R interval before the
blocked P wave, and there is no shortening
of P-R interval after the blocked P wave.

Fig. 14-24. Mobitz type II block.

This is called Mobitz type II block; *it is practically always seen in the presence of preexisting bundle branch block because the AV nodal tissues never behave in this manner.* Very occasionally this type of block may occur within the tissues of the His bundle, but it is the rarest of exceptions when it does.

If first-degree AV block, two-to-one, or other "fixed ratio" blocks appear in the presence of bundle-branch block, the astute cardiologist can often manipulate the sinus rate by speeding and slowing it to see if a true Mobitz II phenomenon can be produced. If it can, the cardiologist can be absolutely certain that the P waves are blocked by failure of conduction in the remaining bundle branch.

Complete heart block

When the ectopic, or reserve, pacemaker driving the ventricles inscribes a narrow QRS complex, it is clear that the site of block must be in the AV node or His bundle because the narrow QRS complexes show that the bundle-branch system is functioning normally. On the other hand, if the ectopic pacemaker inscribes wide QRS complexes (0.12 second wide or more) the ectopic pacemaker on which the patient's life depends may be somewhere in the ventricles below the bifurcation of the bundle-branch system. When the heart is being driven by this kind of ventricular reserve pacemaker, it is very likely that the site of block is in the bundle branches, that is, both bundle branches have failed and by failing have produced complete AV block (Fig. 14-25).

• • •

The rest of this chapter will describe the causes of these types of block, their significance, and their treatment. Before going any further, you are urged to study this glossary of terms and definitions and be quite sure they are all familiar and clearly identified.

Glossary of definitions in atrioventricular block

normal atrioventricular conductions A PR interval of 0.12 to 0.20 second (3 to 5 small squares on the ECG).

normal ventricular activation time A ventricular complex less than 0.11 second in width.

first-degree AV block Each atrial wave traverses the AV conducting system successfully and produces a ventricular response, but takes longer than normal doing so; the PR interval is prolonged.

second-degree AV block
   "fixed ratio" Every other P wave is blocked and every alternate one is conducted to the ventricles. Rarely the ratio may be three to one or four to one.

   Wenckebach block There is progressive fatigue of the cells in the AV node with corresponding progressive prolongation of PR interval until one transmission fails entirely. In the pause after the blocked transmission the cells recover and the next PR interval is again shortened.

   Mobitz type II block There is abrupt block of an occasional P wave *without any warning prolongation of the PR intervals before the blocked P. There*

Complete atrioventricular block in the bundle-branch system

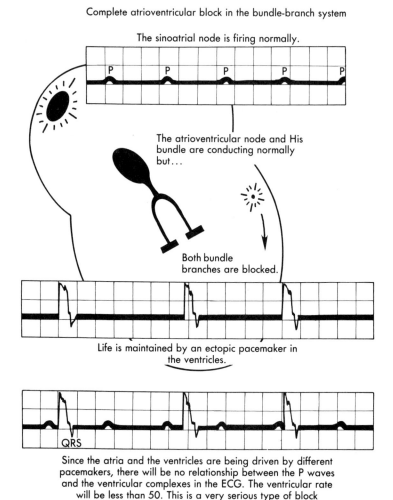

The sinoatrial node is firing normally.

The atrioventricular node and His bundle are conducting normally but...

Both bundle branches are blocked.

Life is maintained by an ectopic pacemaker in the ventricles.

Since the atria and the ventricles are being driven by different pacemakers, there will be no relationship between the P waves and the ventricular complexes in the ECG. The ventricular rate will be less than 50. This is a very serious type of block and practically always requires permanent pacing.

Fig. 14-25. Complete heart block in the bundle-branch system.

is also no recovery of the PR interval after the blocked P wave. This type of block will practically always be seen in the presence of preexisting bundle-branch block, since this abrupt all-or-none conduction is a characteristic of bundle-branch tissue and is never seen in the AV node.

third-degree AV block None of the atrial impulses reach the ventricles; life is maintained by the discharge of an ectopic reserve pacemaker in the AV node-His bundle area or in the ventricles themselves.

pseudo–complete AV block A reserve pacemaker begins firing rapidly, even though there is nothing wrong with the AV conducting system; because this extra pacemaker is firing rapidly, its beats "get in the way of" the normal beats coming down from the sinoatrial node through the AV node and prevent them from reaching the ventricles by discharging the tissues electrically before the normal impulse can traverse them. *Because of this possibility, complete AV block cannot be diagnosed unless the atrioventricular rate is below 50,* at which point it is concluded there is ample time for impulses from the atria to reach the ventricles if the tissues are capable of conducting.

bundle-branch block Block of either bundle branch widens the ventricular complex of 0.12 second or greater because of the prolonged period required for the "backward" invasion of the blocked ventricle.

fascicular block Block of one of the two fascicles of the left bundle branch detected by change in direction of the forces recorded on the electrocardiogram.

bifascicular block Block of the right bundle branch and one of the two fascicles of the left bundle branch.

bilateral bundle-branch block or trifascicular block Complete block of the bundle-branch system producing complete atrioventricular block; this may mean block of the early, or undivided, part of both bundle branches, or it can happen because the right bundle branch is blocked as well as both fascicles of the left.

AV block: causes and treatment
Temporary block in the AV node

First-, second-, or third-degree block may appear in the AV node as a result of drug intoxication. Digitalis, quinidine, beta-blocking drugs (propanolol), procainamide, and certain mood-elevating drugs (tricyclics) can all delay conduction through the AV node. Treatment is withdrawal of drugs and temporary pacing if the heart is dangerously slow.

AV nodal block of any degree may be produced by myocardial infarction, almost always infarction of the right coronary artery. This tends to be a benign type of block and rarely needs more than temporary pacing while the patient is under care in the coronary care unit during the first week of the process. This type of block practically always resolves with resumption of normal conduction two to three weeks after the myocardial infarct, and it is almost unheard of for an inferior myocardial infarct as a result of occlusion of the right coronary artery to produce permanent heart block. Progressive AV nodal block may result from degeneration of the AV nodal tissues as a result of a number of kinds of inflammation of the heart or simply as a part of the aging process. First- or second-degree AV nodal block rarely require more than careful observation unless there are long pauses in the second-degree block that actually produce symptoms. *Clinically significant second-degree AV nodal block is practically always caused by cardiac drugs or by the effect of a myocardial infarction. Spontaneous second-degree AV nodal block is quite rare; spontaneous second-degree AV nodal block severe enough to require pacemaker insertion is even more rare. I don't suppose I have seen more than two or three cases in the last fifteen years.* If second-degree AV nodal block is not temporary (that is, not the result of drugs or a myocardial infarct), if it produces pauses long enough to generate symptoms, and if these pauses can clearly be shown to be the cause of the patient's symptoms, then and only then will pacemaker insertion be justified.

Third-degree AV block as a result of progressive disease may become permanent and may well require insertion of a pacemaker.

Block within the bundle-branch system

For the simple bundle-branch block no therapy is needed beyond observation of the patient.

Bifascicular block (block of the right bundle-branch and one of the divisions of the left)

No therapy is needed for bifascicular block as long as atrioventricular conduction remains normal.

Mobitz type II block

Mobitz type II block almost always indicates failure of conduction in both bundle branches—permanent bundle-branch block on one side and occasional failure on the other. There is a high risk of abrupt cessation of heartbeat with Stokes-Adams attacks; Mobitz type II block is almost always an indication for insertion of a pacemaker.

Complete heart block in the bundle-branch system

Complete heart block with an ectopic ventricular pacemaker, characterized by wide ventricular complexes driving the ventricles, is almost always an indication for pacemaker insertion.

Gray areas

Two-to-one or other "fixed ratio" block with bundle-branch block suggests the possibility of intermittent failure of both bundle branches. The rate should be manipulated to see if a true Mobitz II phenomenon can be produced. Repeated Holter monitors should be recorded to see if there are periods of failure of transmission from atria to ventricles. This kind of investigation becomes much more urgent if the patient is experiencing symptoms of vertigo or syncope. If the patient is completely asymptomatic, feels well, and exercises without untoward effects, nothing more than careful observation is warranted.

Clinical significance of AV block

When atrioventricular block produces long pauses in the heart rhythm, the delivery of blood to the brain, of course, may fall below the minimum needed to maintain full consciousness. Dizziness or fainting will be the two commonest

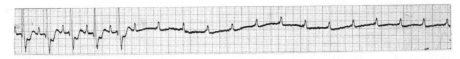

Fig. 14-26. Stokes-Adams seizure. Complete failure of conduction from atria to ventricles with ventricular standstill.

symptoms of this kind of slowing of the heart rate, just as with the sick sinus syndrome.

Atrioventricular block may produce very long pauses in the heart rhythm which can threaten life.

Stokes-Adams attacks. Two Dublin physicians, Stokes and Adams, described episodes of abrupt loss of consciousness when they found a victim stretched on the cobblestone of the streets or the floor of his home, pulseless. What they were describing was an abrupt episode of complete asystole, or stoppage of heartbeat, caused by failure of AV conduction. In the presence of some kinds of heart block conduction from atria to ventricles may suddenly stop for a matter of some seconds, halting the flow of blood to the brain completely and producing abrupt lack of consciousness. This "drop attack," or acute loss of consciousness because of cessation of heartbeat, is called a Stokes-Adams attack.

Stokes-Adams seizures, or loss of consciousness because of failure of the heart to beat for a time, are extremely dangerous and may be fatal. When there is a long period without a heartbeat, brain damage is common. As far as can be determined the first Stokes-Adams seizure is rarely fatal, but the second or third is very likely to be (Fig. 14-26).

The documentation of a true Stokes-Adams seizure, when it can be proved to be a result of atrioventricular block, is beyond any question an indication for pacemaker insertion.

Pacemakers and pacemaker insertion

If the diagnosis of the type of AV block has been made correctly and evaluated properly, the insertion of a pacemaker does not present much of a problem. When block appears in the course of a myocardial infarct, a temporary pacemaker can quickly be threaded from a neck or arm vein into the right ventricle with electrocardiographic or x-ray monitoring. This is often a lifesaving procedure.

Permanent pacemakers (p. 178). The power pack of the permanent pacemaker, which is a small steel, irregular ovoid about half the size of a small doughnut, can be implanted under the skin, most commonly in the upper chest and sometimes in the upper abdomen. In most cases the pacing wires will be threaded from the great veins underneath the collar bone, down through the right atrium and into the right ventricle. The pacing wire is then connected to the power pack and from then on it is a simple matter of letting a rather small wound heal.

The commonest kind of pacemaker used today is the ventricular demand pacemaker; that is, a pacemaker placed in the right ventricle, connected to a set of circuits that permit it to fire only when the normal heartbeat does not arrive on time. Thus this kind of pacemaker fires "on demand."

In certain rare situations when the output of the heart is seriously jeopardized or when the ventricular pacemaker has created some problems by retrograde conduction up through the atria, an atrioventricular sequential pacemaker may be inserted. This is a pacemaker that has two electrodes, one in the right atrium and one in the right ventricle, and a more complex set of circuits that fire the two chambers in sequence just as if they were being activated by the normal impulse from the sinus node.

The atrioventricular sequential pacemaker is more expensive and more complicated than the simple ventricular demand one, and hence it is not used in most cases. However, in properly selected cases this kind of pacemaker can be extremely useful.

Complications of permanent ventricular pacing include perforation of the ventricle by the pacemaker tip, infection (endocarditis) around the pacemaker wire, formation of blood clot somewhere along the course of the pacemaker wire, and in a series of cases I am studying at this time, deformity of the tricuspid valve because of the presence of the foreign body, that is, the pacemaker wire exerting pressure against one of the leaflets of the valve. The pacemaker wire may break and part of it may float on into the lungs or "backward" into the veins of the brain or the body: this can be a catastrophe.

•   •   •

This chapter has been long and very detailed for good reasons. Pacemaker therapy has been one of the great advances of twentieth century cardiology; many patients are alive today because pacemakers have been available. *On the other hand, the overutilization of pacemakers has reach very serious proportions on a national scale, and the only real remedy to this seems to be thorough education of patients about the kind of diseases that slow the heartbeat and the precise types of abnormal conduction of the electrical impulse of the heartbeat that justify insertion of a pacemaker.*

ELECTROPHYSIOLOGIC STUDIES

Now and then a rare case appears when a patient reports serious symptoms such as outright fainting and the electrocardiogram reveals block of one bundle branch without any recorded failure of conduction from atria to ventricles. If after extended investigation in such a case no other cause for the fainting can be found, and if repeated electrocardiographic studies with changes of rate and prolonged observation do not reveal any evidence of atrioventricular block, the performance of a special kind of study called a His bundle recording may be justified.

When the electric impulse passes through the bundle of His, an electric signal can be recorded if a catheter is threaded into the right side of the heart so that recording electrodes are placed close to the His bundle. By taking records from other electrodes in the atria, from those at the His bundle site, and in the ventricle, the cardiologist can measure the exact time required for passage of the electric impulse from atria to His bundle and from the His bundle into the upper bundle-branch system (Fig. 14-27).

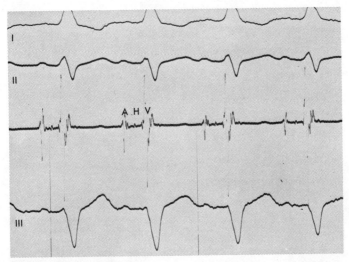

Heart rate: 108 50 mse H-V: 50 msec

Fig. 14-27. His bundle study.

The normal time required for an impulse to pass from the His bundle to the bundle-branch system has been established; it is called the His-to-ventricle time, or HV time. Some researchers think that if one bundle branch is already blocked and the HV time is prolonged on the other side (the side that is still functioning), there is an increased risk of the appearance of some kind of block in the remaining functioning bundle branch with failure of atrioventricular conduction. For this reason, they argue, if the patient is having fainting spells that cannot otherwise be accounted for, the finding of bundle-branch block with prolonged HV time may justify implantation of a pacemaker, even though actual failure of atrioventricular conduction has not been documented. Other equally competent researchers argue that the finding of a prolonged HV time in this setting is meaningless; in their series of patients they find the same likelihood of going into some kind of atrioventricular block regardless of the HV measurements. The whole subject is a matter for research.

The leading authorities on cardiac arrhythmias are substantially agreed that the necessary information for most practical diagnoses can be obtained from the ordinary electrocardiogram or the Holter monitor recording; recording of the His-bundle potential, they agree, is a splendid research tool which has given much basic information, but it is very rarely needed in practical clinical diagnosis.

From the data I can gather around the country it appears that in some areas His-bundle recordings are being performed enthusiastically and with little justification. Since the procedure does involve catheterization of the heart with a good deal of expense and some risk, it should be undertaken only after prolonged and careful consultation. Patients or other physicians have often called me to ask about the appropriateness of a suggested His-bundle recording; my usual answer, if the patient lives in another city, is that they try to find a cardiologist who knows more about

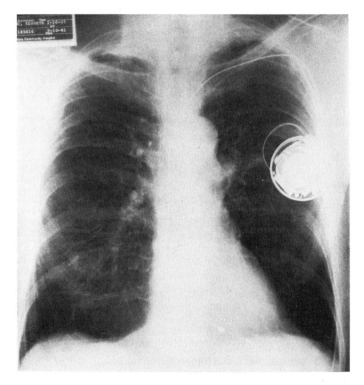

Fig. 14-28. X-ray film showing pacemaker in place under the skin of the chest wall. The pacer tip can be seen in the bottom of the heart shadow.

cardiac arrhythmias and electrocardiography. The chances are that the procedure won't be necessary.

His-bundle recording may be useful with some rare rapid rhythms of the heart when the physician cannot be sure if the ectopic firing is coming from the atria, the junction, or the ventricles. This, again, should be extremely rare. Before permitting this kind of expensive invasion of the heart the patient should insist on consultation, since it is likely that a cardiologist with special skills in arrhythmias might be able to make the diagnosis from the surface electrocardiogram.

QUESTIONS FOR THE PATIENT WITH SICK SINUS SYNDROME

1. What type of sick sinus syndrome is present? If it is the bradycardia, or slow, type, what form does it take? Is sinoatrial exit block present? Are there frequent sinus pauses? Is simple bradycardia the problem? If so, how long are the pauses and how slow is the bradycardia?
2. If the bradycardia-tachycardia syndrome is diagnosed, what type of tachycardia is present? How does the sinus node function between

Guidelines for permanent pacemaker implantations*

Complete heart block, acquired

Congenital complete heart block, symptomatic†

Mobitz type II block (nonconducted P waves with fixed PR interval before and after nonconducted P waves, generally with prolonged QRS complexes)

Bifascicular block (RBBB‡ and LAH‡) and syncopal spells not due to other central nervous system or vascular disorder

Incomplete trifascicular block (RBBB,‡ LAH,‡ HV interval,‡ 65) if

1. New and permanent after acute myocardial infarct even if asymptomatic—may be indicated
2. Bradycardia-tachycardia syndrome, symptomatic† or requiring the use of digitalis or propranolol
3. Atrial fibrillation with slow ventricular rate, less than 50 beats per minute, symptomatic

Carotid sinus hypersensitivity

Overdrive for arrhythmia control

---

*Recommendations of a committee reported in the Journal of the American Medical Association, August 14, 1981. Dr. Atul B. Chokshi, Dr. Howard S. Friedman, Dr. Monte Malach, Dr. Balendu C. Vasavada, and Dr. Sheldon J. Bleicher. These guidelines were drawn up by a committee of cardiologists and cardiac surgeons to review the adequacy of pacemaker insertions at a large teaching center. They certainly represent reasonable criteria, although cardiologists might differ over some minor definitions and distinctions.

†Dizziness, syncope, confusion, angina pectoris, heart failure at the time of arrhythmia, or conduction disturbance.

‡RBBB, right bundle-branch block; LAH, left anterior hemiblock; HV, His-ventricular.

---

bouts of rapid beating, and how has it been documented that the sinus node is functioning subnormally?

3. Is the abnormal sinus node behavior the result of drug treatment? Many common drugs can slow the sinus node, producing an artificial sick sinus sundrome—digitalis, quinidine, propranolol and other beta-blocking drugs, procainamide, and certain drugs used for control of nervous states, chiefly the antidepressant drugs called tricyclics. Is the physician sure that there were no such drugs circulating in the body when the observations documenting the presence of sick sinus syndrome were made?

4. Have adequate Holter recordings and other electrocardiographic tracings been obtained to prove that the subnormal sinus node function is really the cause of the symptoms? In other words, was there really a demonstration of a period of some kind of sinus node slowing with

Indications for permanent pacemaking*

    I. Complete heart block
   II. Mobitz type II block demonstrated on ECG at rest or during exercise or during a Holter monitor recording
  III. AV nodal block of high degree, producing periods of asystole that are symptomatic
      A. The block is not drug induced
      B. The block is not a manifestation of transient ischemia (i.e., during myocardial infarction)
  IV. Sick sinus syndrome with periods of asystole clearly documented by ECG recording to correlate with symptoms of severe vertigo or syncope or to facilitate medication treatment of tachy-arrhythmias.

Comment: To these should be added the following:

   V. Carotid sinus hypersensitivity (Patients who have a very sensitive carotid sinus with stimulation of the vagal nerve on slight motion of the head or neck and periods of complete block as a result.)
  VI. Overdrive for arrhythmia control (In rare cases of rapid heart beat special kind of pacemaker can be inserted to "overdrive" and thus control the arrhythmia.)
 VII. Bifascicular block (right bundle-branch block plus left anterior hemiblock) with syncopal spells that have been carefully investigated (It is assumed that disorders of the central nervous system or the peripheral vascular system have been ruled out as causes. Supporting documentation may include prolonged HV interval.)

*Prepared by Southern Arizona PSRO.

significant pauses in the heart rate at the same time the patient noted dizziness or faintness?

5. Has an adequate search been made for other causes of dizziness or fainting? It's important to remember that most dizziness and fainting is *not* caused by any abnormality of heart rhythm.
6. Is the pacemaker being inserted simply because a slow heart rate was recorded during sleep? The heart responds to the body's needs through a number of "thermostat" or feedback mechanisms. During sleep when the body's needs are low, the heart rate commonly falls into the 40s or even lower without any harmful effect. This nighttime slowing has sometimes been used to justify pacemaker insertion when, in fact, it is a normal phenomenon.

7. Is the diagnosis of sick sinus syndrome based only on electrophysiologic studies? There have been many attempts to evaluate sinus node function by electrically driving the sinus node through a temporary pacing wire threaded into the right atrium. By observing how long it takes for the sinus node to recover its function after a period of rapid artificial beating and by making other observations it is sometimes possible to get a general idea of sinus node function, but these studies really do not correlate very well with the actual diagnosis of sick sinus syndrome. They are useful only as a help to make a decision in very difficult "gray-area" cases. They are not a substitute for actual observation and demonstration of subnormal sinus node function under normal living conditions.

QUESTIONS FOR THE PATIENT WITH AV BLOCK

1. Do I have second-degree block or complete AV block? (If he tells you that you only have first-degree heart block, ask for a consultant.)
2. If I have second-degree block, is it in the AV node? Is it Wenckebach block? How slow is the slowest heart rate you have recorded? Is this abnormally slow rate actually causing my symptoms? (Ask for consultation whenever a permanent pacemaker is proposed for second-degree block localized in the AV node. A pacemaker is rarely needed in this condition.)
3. Is the second-degree block in the bundle-branch system? How do you know?
4. Do I have Mobitz II block? If so, do I have preexisting bundle-branch block? (If Mobitz type II block is alleged without bundle-branch block, ask for consultation; this is urgent.)
5. Do I have bifascicular block; that is, right bundle-branch block and block of one fascicle of the left bundle? Is there some evidence of actual delay or failure of AV conduction associated with this bifascicular block? (If bifascicular block alone is proposed as a reason for a pacemaker, consultation is urgent.)
6. Do I have complete AV block? If so, is it in the AV node or in the bundle branch system? If so—
7. Is the ventricular rate under 50? (If it isn't, consultation is urgent; nobody can really make a diagnosis of complete heart block if the ventricular rate is over 50.)
8. Is this a permanent state? Is it intermittent, appearing only occasionally, or is it predictably temporary?
9. If temporary or intermittent, is the block caused by medications that I'm taking? Isn't there a chance that it will stop if they were cut down or eliminated?
10. Is it caused by some temporary disease such as ischemia or inflammation, which may improve or disappear?

15 Pregnancy and heart disease

This chapter will be blunt, direct, and sometimes grim. Pregnancy with heart disease is that kind of subject. Usually the physician reassures, comforts, and encourages. There are times when he must be direct and must present frightening facts as truthfully as possible. A pregnant woman with a diseased heart does not need a fatherly pat on the shoulder and a chirp of encouragement. She needs the truth.

Even before physicians knew much about heart disease they knew that pregnancy and heart disease made a bad combination. They had watched women with various types of heart disease throughout pregnancy; they had learned that these women often were in trouble toward the end of the pregnancy. They also learned that many of these women died of congestive heart failure or of other complications related to their heart disease. They knew that even after the baby was delivered the woman was still in considerable danger and might well die of her heart disease.

Physicians now know quite accurately why pregnancy is dangerous for women with heart disease. Physicians know with fair accuracy which patients with heart disease can safely go through pregnancy and which cannot.

Some women with heart disease can carry a pregnancy and deliver a child with no danger or difficulty. Other women with heart disease face a risk so severe that they should never become pregnant in the first place and should not be allowed to carry the pregnancy to completion if they do. This chapter will explain why pregnancy is bad for women with serious heart disease and just what the risks are. It will further try to explain how the physician can decide which woman with heart disease can safely carry a pregnancy and which one cannot.

As far as the heart is concerned, the most important thing that happens during pregnancy *is a rise in the total volume of blood.* This increase in blood volume starts in the first three months of pregnancy. It increases steadily; in the ninth lunar month the increase in blood volume is about 45% in the average woman. The heart must pump a total volume of blood that is almost half again as great as it was before pregnancy started. Obviously this is an extra work load for the heart. In cardiac terms the woman is walking up a gradually sloping mountain throughout her pregnancy.

At the peak load of pregnancy oxygen consumption by the body is up 25%. The heart pumps 10% to 20% more blood with each beat; this means that the total output of the heart per minute or per hour will be up about 50%. The increase in work load is gradual during the first three or four months of pregnancy; it becomes much more severe in the sixth, seventh, and eighth months and then tapers off somewhat during the last month before delivery.

Other abnormalities of blood flow help to load the heart. The placenta, which nourishes the embryo, probably acts as a shunt, or arteriovenous fistula.

This means that blood runs from a fairly large artery to a fairly large vein without ever going through a capillary bed. Whenever a fistula of this kind exists, it throws a load on the circulation. Many researchers believe that the blood vessel connections in the placenta are just a direct shunt from artery to vein. This may be one of the reasons for the increased work load on the heart during pregnancy.

There is much **dilution** of the blood during pregnancy; the liquid, or plasma, part of the blood rises without an equivalent rise in blood cells or oxygen carrying part of the blood. For this reason, most pregnant women appear to be anemic during the middle and last parts of their pregnancy.

The mass of the infant's body and its surrounding fluids act as a block to blood flow from the veins of the legs to the upper body. This is simple pressure. The effect is the same as if you were to grip your fingers around the middle of your forearm and squeeze until the veins in the hands stood out. Back pressure in the veins of the lower legs tends to dilate these vessels, which further complicates the already abnormal pattern of blood flow.

Normal women adjust easily to this increased work load. There will rarely be any difficulty except for some swelling in the ankles caused by back pressure in the veins. Normally, the heart will increase its output of blood per beat and will thus propel the increased volume of fluid.

The woman with a diseased heart, however, may be caught in a dangerous trap. If the heart disease is severe, the heart may not be able to increase its output, and it may not be able to pump more blood per minute than it is already pumping. The heart will then fail in the face of the huge increase in volume of blood to be pumped.

Total load increase on the heart is not very great until about the sixth month of pregnancy. Many women with heart disease will find that the first three, four or five months of pregnancy are uneventful. In the sixth, seventh, and eighth months, many such women will suddenly find that they are in trouble. Breathing becomes difficult, the heart pounds and races, and the patient is exhausted on slight exertion. She now finds that walking about the house or climbing a single flight of stairs may produce frightening shortness of breath, so that she must sit down and rest. Congestive heart failure, which should now be familiar to readers of this book, has begun its work. In this case the causative agent is going to be right on hand, producing more trouble for another three months. The increased volume of blood will still be present and must be pumped until the woman has delivered the baby no matter what measures are taken. The pregnant woman with heart disease is like a woman climbing a tremendously long flight of stairs twenty-four hours a day with no chance of stopping throughout the last three months of pregnancy.

How many women with heart disease can survive? How dangerous is pregnancy and delivery in a woman with heart disease? Which patients should undertake pregnancy and which should not? To answer these questions, the reader must understand the functional classification of heart disease. This useful index was devised by the New York Heart Association; it is used universally by cardiologists.

Functional grade one. This grade includes patients who have heart disease but who can carry out any ordinary and even most heavy activities without symptoms or difficulty. These patients have no limitation on physical capability.

Functional grade two. This includes heart patients who can carry out ordinary physical activity such as walking, light athletics, and the work of most day-by-day occupations in our society. However, extraordinary exertions such as mountain climbing, strenuous athletics, running, and the like will produce difficulty and must be avoided.

Functional grade three. This group experiences difficulty such as shortness of breath or pain even during light to moderate activity. A woman carrying bundles from the supermarket to her car, a man walking eight blocks from his home to work, or a golfer strolling about the links would notice some limitation of activity because of heart disease.

Functional grade four. This is the most seriously ill group; these patients feel symptoms such as pain or shortness of breath even at rest in a chair or bed.

With this functional index as a guide, the physician can choose those patients who can safely approach pregnancy most of the time. Women in functional grade one need have no fear of childbearing. They can produce large families with no more risk than their sisters without heart disease. Women in functional grade two have much the same outlook. They, too, can carry children and go through labor with almost no increase in risk. Functional grade two is a large grade. There are subdivisions within it. Just what is meant by **strenuous** and **moderate** activity will differ with different individuals. A woman who is somewhere on the borderline between functional grade two and grade three will be evaluated differently from a woman who is somewhere on the borderline between functional grade one and grade two. The women in functional grade three should not become pregnant. Some of them will be able to carry a child and will survive delivery. However, an alarming large percentage will not. All patients in this group can expect to have severe problems with their heart in the last three months of pregnancy; they may well go into congestive heart failure during this time, during labor, or during the dangerous forty-eight hours after delivery. Patients in functional grade four should never, under any circumstances, become pregnant, and if they do, they should never be allowed to carry the pregnancy to term. The chances of death in functional grade four patients who become pregnant are overwhelming. Their chances of carrying a pregnancy safely are so small that they are not acceptable in medical or ethical terms.

What specific dangers does a woman face who goes through pregnancy with serious heart disease? (**Serious heart disease** means functional grade three or four for purposes of this discussion.) She is almost sure to go into some degree of congestive heart failure during the last part of her pregnancy. The strain of labor throws an additional severe load on the heart, and many women go into a kind of heart failure that does not respond well to medical management during labor and delivery. After the placenta has separated from the uterus, the pattern of blood flow in the body changes drastically. For this and other reasons, the forty-eight hours after delivery are very dangerous in women with serious heart disease. To reiterate, *cardiac patients in functional grades three or four will almost certainly go into congestive heart failure at some time during the latter portion of pregnancy, during labor, or following delivery. A woman who has had some kind of congestive failure before pregnancy is absolutely certain to go into congestive heart failure during her pregnancy.* Many times this congestive failure does not respond to medical management. It may be fatal. Other complications associated with heart disease are common in pregnant women. Blood clots in the lung, or pulmonary emboli, account for about 15% of all deaths in this group. Shock and hemorrhage are also important dangers. Shock and hemorrhage are more common and more dangerous in women with heart disease than in healthy women. Subacute bacterial endocarditis, which is an infection of the heart lining, is still another hazard.

The woman who is in severe grade three or grade four functional state faces a greater risk going through a pregnancy than she would if she were a mountain climber attacking Mt. Everest. The picture is grim. However, it is not as grim as it was. Improved methods of medical treatment and improved means of diagnosis have changed the statistics in favor of the prospective mother. Patients who formerly would have been thought hopeless can now be carried through a pregnancy successfully with the combined efforts of the cardiologist, the obstetrician, and the family physician. In any of these cases, however, intensive medical care and supervision are necessary if the patient is to be given a chance of healthy survival.

What of the infant in all this discussion? Statistics here are discouraging. In the functional grade three to four group the infant death rate is four times that of children delivered of mothers without heart disease.

Again we ask the question, "What patient with heart disease should carry a pregnancy?" There is no single answer that will apply to all patients. A woman who has had no children may be willing to face a greater risk to achieve the fulfillment of childbirth. A woman who has had a large family and who has suffered increasing cardiac difficulty with each birth will certainly be a different problem. The woman who has actually been in congestive failure presents no problem at all. She should never get pregnant, and her pregnancy should be interrupted if she does. The patient, her husband, and the physician must sit down and weigh all these factors. They must consider first the woman's cardiac state and her chances of surviving pregnancy and labor. They must consider next the couple's desire for a child and their position with respect to their family. They must also consider religious convictions that may bear on the problem. Above all, the odds must be viewed in a completely realistic manner, with no glossing over and no attempt to paint a rosy picture. After considering all this, if the patient and her physician decided to proceed with her pregnancy, modern medical science can at least guarantee that her chances are many times better than they were twenty years ago.

What kinds of heart disease do pregnant women usually have? Valvular heart disease is the greatest menace that threatens the pregnant cardiac patient. Congenital heart disease is rare, and today it is frequently corrected by surgery before a woman reaches the childbearing age. Hypertensive heart disease is relatively rare in women in the childbearing age. Rheumatic scarring of the mitral and aortic valves accounts for 96% or more of all cases of heart disease complicated by pregnancy.

Rheumatic fever poses a further threat. If a woman has had a recent attack of rheumatic fever, there is the possibility that some of the rheumatic nodules may still be "smoldering" in the heart muscle. The rheumatic fever may still be quietly following an insidious, hidden course. If this is true, the pregnancy will make the woman a great deal worse and may very well end in a disaster. For this reason, pregnancy in anyone who has recently had rheumatic fever is to be avoided at all costs.

What if the patient and the physician decide that the pregnancy should be interrupted? I hasten to point out that there are those whose religious scruples will bring a different light to bear on the problem. This book does not intend to become involved in theological questions; I leave those for the patient to decide with her clergyman and her family.

Assuming that the mother's life is the first consideration, it is safe to say that all patients in a functional grade four state and the majority of patients in a functional grade three state should have pregnancy interrupted by surgical removal of the fetus. This can be done safely during the first three months of the pregnancy. After this, abdominal operation is needed, and the risk is greatly increased. Interruption of a pregnancy by curettement during the first three months is a very simple and safe procedure in skilled hands. The point to be emphasized is this: the woman with heart disease who becomes pregnant must make her condition known at once. I have seen tragic results of inexplicable delaying and hesitance by pregnant women who were perfectly well aware of their condition and who were equally aware of their serious heart disease. If steps are to be taken to save the patient's life, they had best be taken in the first three months.

What of the pregnant cardiac patient who survives pregnancy, labor, and the period immediately after childbirth? This is a hotly argued point by physicians. Some authorities insist that these women show the effects of strain on their heart during the five years or so following childbirth. They point out that a large number of these women go into congestive heart failure during this period, with an alarming percentage of deaths. There are many figures to back this point of view.

On the other hand, other authorities with equally large number of figures insist that this is not true. They maintain that women follow what would have been the natural course of their heart disease anyway. They believe that the woman who survives childbirth does not suffer any increased risk and that her cardiac status does not deteriorate. It is not possible to give a definite answer to this question at this time. I find it difficult to imagine that the prolonged overload of pregnancy would not have a bad long-term effect on any seriously diseased heart.

Heart surgery has changed the menace of pregnancy for many cardiac patients. If a woman has some kind of heart disease that can be corrected by surgery, she can undergo the operation during the early part of her pregnancy with no extra risk. With a more nearly normal heart, she can then go on to a reasonably safe pregnancy and delivery. As surgical techniques improve and as more types of heart disease become surgically curable, the number of women with heart disease who can carry a pregnancy safely is certainly going to increase.

There is another face to this coin; if a woman with heart disease has had surgery, such as correction of mitral stenosis, she should not become pregnant for at least a year after completion of the surgery.

To sum up this whole chapter, one can say that the woman with heart disease who becomes pregnant faces a risk. The seriousness of the heart disease present is the factor that determines just how great this risk will be. The physician can usually make a reasonable estimate of the risk in a particular case; the crucial decision then lies in the hands of the patient and her husband. They must weigh the social, personal, and religious factors that they believe are important and must proceed accordingly.

Remember that prevention of infectious endocarditis is crucial during and after delivery; the usual prophylactic antibiotics should be administered to any woman with known valvular heart disease before, during, and after delivery.

The last word in this chapter will be encouraging: modern medical advances have made it possible to bring many women with heart disease through childbirth with safety and without apparent serious injury to their heart. This is true of cases that would have been considered hopeless in years gone by. Cardiac surgery is making it possible for women with heart disease to go through pregnancy and labor almost as safely as their healthy sisters. Pregnancy in heart disease has been a ''dark continent'' in the medical world. It is a continent that is growing brighter with every year that passes.

QUESTIONS FOR THE PREGNANT PATIENT WITH HEART DISEASE AND HER PHYSICIANS

1. What exactly is wrong with my heart?
2. Do I have disease of the heart valves or the heart muscle?
3. What functional grade do I fall into in terms of the New York Heart Association classification?
4. What is likely to happen to my cardiac function during the rest of pregnancy when the increased blood volume exerts its effect?
5. What is the risk at the time of delivery and immediately afterward?
6. Should I have corrective surgery for my heart problem early in the pregnancy?
7. Is the risk of sickness or death from my heart disease greater than the risk to the fetus from corrective surgery?
8. What would be the effect on my heart in years to come if I continue this pregnancy, considering that I have heart disease?
9. Shouldn't I be on endocarditis prophylaxis at the time of delivery?
10. What effect will my heart disease have on my unborn child during this pregnancy?

16 Congenital heart disease

Out of every thousand people you meet walking down the street it is likely that ten or twelve will have been born with some abnormality of the structure of the heart. In other words, their hearts were simply "put together" incorrectly, with holes where there should be walls or with great vessels leading out of the wrong chambers. There are a great many different types of congenital structural abnormalities of the heart, and some of them are extremely complicated. It would not be reasonable for you to attempt to learn all about this very technical subject, but, on the other hand, since one out of every hundred people probably has some congenital abnormality, it is worthwhile to explain the most common types and to alert the possible patient to some danger signs and to some necessary medical precautions.

CONNECTIONS BETWEEN THE PULMONARY CIRCULATION AND THE GENERAL CIRCULATION

The part of the circulatory system that includes the right heart, the pulmonary arteries, and the pulmonary veins is often referred to as the "pulmonary circulation," or "the lesser circulation," since it is a relatively small set of structures. It is also a low-pressure system (Chapter 2). The part of the circulatory system that starts with the left heart and continues out through the aorta, through all the vessels of the body, and back through the veins to the right heart is called the "greater circulation," simply because it is a great deal larger in actual dimensions. It is also a high-pressure system. An average blood pressure in the aorta will be about 120/80, whereas an average blood pressure in the pulmonary artery will be approximately one fifth that much, or about 24/12.

Normally, there is no connection between the pulmonary circulation and the greater circulation; you will remember that there is a watertight septum between the two sides of the heart, and the blood moves from the right side of the heart to the left side by way of the lungs.

One of the commonest groups of congenital abnormalities of the heart is characterized by a hole, or leak, that permits blood to move directly through the septum of the heart, thus creating a new and abnormal kind of circuit.

Atrial septal defect (Fig. 16-1)

A persistent hole in the septum between the two atria is referred to as an atrial septal defect; blood will flow through this hole, usually from the left atrium to the right atrium, thence to the right ventricle and back around to the lungs. In other words, some of the blood that should be going on into the left ventricle and out to the body is being recirculated back through the right side of the heart and into the lungs again. With a large hole in the septum, the volume of blood being

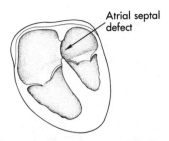

Fig. 16-1. Atrial septal defect. The hole between the atria permits flow of blood from the left atrium to right atrium and then to the right ventricle and around again through the lungs.

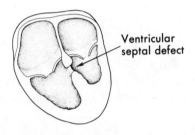

Fig. 16-2. Ventricular septal defect. Blood flows from the left ventricle to the right ventricle and is recirculated through the lungs.

pumped into the lungs may be two or three times as great as the volume being pumped on out to the body.

Ventricular septal defect (Fig. 16-2)

The same kind of hole, or defect, may be present in the septum between the ventricles. About the same thing will happen; that is, blood will be pumped from the left ventricle back through the septal defect into the right ventricle and around again through the lungs. Again the pulmonary circuit will be "overloaded" with blood, sometimes in very large volume.

Patent ductus arteriosus (Fig. 16-3)

When the baby is in the womb floating in liquid, of course it cannot breathe. It depends on the mother's blood for its oxygen. For this reason, during fetal life the lungs are short-circuited and there is a connection directly between the pulmonary artery and the aorta whereby the oxygenated blood provided by the mother can circulate through the baby's body. This connection is called a ductus arteriosus. Normally it disappears about two weeks after birth, but sometimes it persists throughout life. If the ductus is large, there is, again, a shunt between the greater circulation and the lesser, or pulmonary, circulation; this time the blood pumped out of the left ventricle into the aorta recirculates back through the ductus into the pulmonary artery. Again, there is a greatly increased volume of

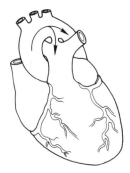

Fig. 16-3. Patent ductus arteriosis. This persistent fetal abnormality permits blood to flow from the aorta into the pulmonary artery where it recirculates through the lungs.

blood pouring from the high-pressure aorta to the low-pressure pulmonary artery, thence through the lungs. With a large ductus, just as with a large atrial or ventricular septal defect, the volume of blood pouring into the lungs may be two or three times as great as the volume of blood being pumped out to the body.

Dangers

Simple, or "secundum" atrial septal defect, unless it is very large, is not immediately dangerous; if the hole is confined to the septum between the atria, the patient can often live into adult life, even into the 40s, 50s, and 60s, before symptoms appear. At that time the increased flow into the lungs may produce a rise in pressure in the rather fragile arteries of the pulmonary system, and the patient will begin to notice pain like angina pectoris, shortness of breath, and vague, generalized fatigability and weakness. At this stage surgery to close the defect is certainly advisable; it is not particularly risky, and results are excellent. If the atrial septal defect is large and reaches down into the septum between the ventricles, the patient will have symptoms at a much earlier age, and surgery should be resorted to in childhood as a rule.

It is easy to diagnose atrial septal defect and differentiate the two types, that is, the mild type, with a hole simply between the two artria, and the more complicated type, with a hole that extends down into the wall between the ventricles. A competent cardiologist using a stethoscope, electrocardiogram, and x-ray examination of the chest can make about 99% of the diagnoses in his office.

The ventricular septal defect and the patent ductus represent a much more serious problem. If the flow into the lungs is large, that is, over twice as large as the flow out to the body, a very dangerous complication may follow. The flow is from a high-pressure system to a low-pressure system—from the left ventricle, or the aorta, into the right ventricle, or the pulmonary artery, and as a result it will be rapid and turbulent. The pulmonary arteries and their branches are simply not designed to handle this kind of high-volume, high-velocity flow, and after a few years the vessels begin to react by thickening their walls. A particular kind of "hardening of the arteries" takes place in the small vessels throughout the pul-

Normal aortic valve viewed
from above

Stenotic, bicuspid
aortic valve

Fig. 16-4. Congenital aortic stenosis. This is a rather common lesion occurring in about one out of every thousand people in the general population.

monary bed, and after a time this becomes irreversible. The pressure in the pulmonary circuit rises until it equals the pressure in the general circulation; at this point the flow, which has been from general circulation to pulmonary circulation, will start to reverse itself and go from pulmonary circuit to general circuit. This means that the lungs are being shut out of the circulation as the blood flows from the right ventricle, or the pulmonary artery, into the left ventricle, or aorta, before it ever has a chance to pick up any oxygen. The patient will begin to become blue (cyanotic). By this time it is too late to do anything to help the patient very much; the changes that have taken place in the small vessels in the pulmonary bed are there to stay, and progressive decline and early death are now inevitable.

Any patient with a patent ductus arteriosus or ventricular septal defect should have careful study early in life to see exactly how large the hole is between the general circulation and the pulmonary circulation; if the flow through the hole is significant, the communication should be closed. By closing the abnormal communication, it is now clear, the fatal complication of pulmonary hypertension and reversal of flow can be totally prevented.

This phenomenon of build up of high pressures in the pulmonary circuit because of rapid, turbulent flow entering it from the general circulation is called Eisenmenger's syndrome. It is a totally preventable disease and is a complication chiefly of the ventricular septal defect and the patent ductus arteriosus that have not been recognized or treated properly.

STENOSIS OF THE SEMILUNAR VALVES (Fig. 16-4)

A child may be born with narrowing—stenosis—of either the pulmonic or aortic valves. Recent studies have shown that a congenital abnormality of the aortic valve is surprisingly common; patients with this abnormality have two flaps, or cusps, instead of the usual three. About 60% of the time this abnormality of the aortic valve does not cause any trouble, and the patient can live out a normal lifetime with one simple precaution. Forty percent of these patients will go on to calcification and degeneration of the valve with significant narrowing in older life so that surgery will be necessary. The congenital bicuspid valve is often characterized by a peculiar clicking noise when it opens, which makes it relatively easy to recognize simply with a stethoscope.

Patients with stenosis of either semilunar valve should receive prophylaxis for bacterial endocarditis whenever they undergo a surgical procedure of an infected or potentially infected cavity.

Pulmonic stenosis

Stenosis of the pulmonic valve is for practical purposes always congenital; rheumatic fever very rarely affects this valve. The narrowing may be so mild that nothing need be done about it throughout a normal lifetime; on the other hand, with severe pulmonic stenosis, the patient will often begin to notice symptoms in childhood or early adult life. I have seen several 16-year-old youngsters brought to me for evaluation of faintness or giddiness appearing during strenuous athletics They always had a murmur that was detected in early childhood, but the mother had usually been reassured that this was "the kind of murmur the child would outgrow." When pulmonic stenosis is severe it cuts down bloodflow to the lungs and during times of greatly increased need the patient will feel exactly the same symptoms that one might feel with aortic stenosis; that is, dizziness or actual fainting. When pulmonic stenosis reaches this stage it is time for surgery, since there is a significant risk of sudden death. A skilled cardiologist can usually make the diagnosis of pulmonic stenosis with a stethoscope, an electrocardiogram, and a chest x-ray plate. Cardiac catheterization is needed prior to surgery, of course, to document the exact severity of the process and possibly to detect other congenital abnormalities that might be associated with it.

Endocarditis prophylaxis is as important here as in the case of aortic stenosis.

TETRALOGY OF FALLOT

This rather exotic name applies to a combination of two of the kinds of defects described so far; Fallot, a famous French cardiologist, described this abnormality, and since it has four elements, he called it a tetralogy. Basically it consists of a large ventricular septal defect combined with some form of pulmonic outflow obstruction, or pulmonic stenosis. If the pulmonic stenosis is severe, of course, the pressure in the right ventricle will be very high and the flow through the ventricular septal defect will be from right ventricle to left ventricle and thence out to the body. This means that the lungs are being "short-circuited," and the blood moving from right ventricle to left ventricle is not picking up any oxygen. As a result the patient may be "blue" or cyanotic. There is an abnormal relationship of the two great vessels to the ventricles in this syndrome, so that a certain amount of blood from the right ventricle is ejected directly into the aorta, thus contributing to the short-circuiting of the lungs and increasing the likelihood of unoxygenated right ventricular blood reaching the tissues of the body (Fig. 16-5).

Tetralogy of Fallot may be extremely mild if there is a small hole between the ventricles and a minimal degree of pulmonic stenosis. These cases will require nothing beyond observation and endocarditis prophylaxis. On the other hand, when it is severe, surgery must be undertaken early. Completely corrective surgery is now available with very good results.

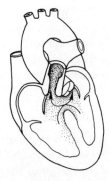

Fig. 16-5. Tetralogy of Fallot. The commonest of the complex congenital arrhythmias, combining a ventricular septal defect with obstruction to flow out of the right ventricle through the pulmonary artery.

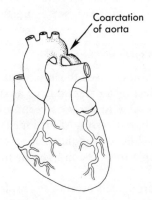

Coarctation
of aorta

Fig. 16-6. Coarctation of the aorta. Narrowing of the aorta severely restricting the flow of blood to the lower parts of the body.

COARCTATION OF THE AORTA

I always warn my interns and residents to look for this congenital abnormality when a young person presents with high blood pressure. Coarctation means narrowing; this kind of narrowing of the aorta may be extreme, so that the great vessel narrows from a structure the size of a generous garden hose down to something about the size of a small piece of twine. The narrowing very commonly takes place near the site of the old ductus arteriosus connection between aorta and pulmonary artery (Fig. 16-6). The effect of this kind of narrowing is perfectly predictable; "upstream" from the narrow area in the aorta the blood pressure will be extremely high; below it the pressure will be abnormally low. A typical patient with coarctation of the aorta might have a pressure of 180/120 in the arms and hardly any detectable pulses in the lower extremities.

The finding of a high blood pressure in one or both arms and very faint or absent pulses in the lower extremities alerts the physician to the possibility of a coarctation at once. The murmur of coarctation is also very helpful and taken together with other findings may be diagnostic.

Surgery for coarctation gives excellent results and the high blood pressure associated with it is generally completely reversible.

COMPLEX CONGENITAL ABNORMALITIES

There are many more complicated kinds of congenital abnormality of the heart that do not warrant presentation here. Sometimes the great vessels are completely reversed so that the aorta comes out of the right ventricle and the pulmonary artery comes out of the left. In these cases unless there is some kind of communication between the two circulations the child will not live long; emergency surgery is frequently necessary. Sometimes children are born with a single ventricle, and sometimes they are born with complete closure of a valve such as the tricuspid valve so that no blood can move forward through it.

In many of these cases competent, swift surgical intervention is called for.

GENERAL OBSERVATIONS

1. Any large connection between the lesser and greater circulations (a ventricular septal defect or a patent ductus arteriosus) should be carefully monitored with a view to early correction before irreversible change takes place in the blood vessels of the lungs. For this reason, persistent heart murmurs in children should be checked by a competent cardiologist, since it is tragic for a lesion like this to progress past a "point of no return."
2. All congenital heart defects except for simple atrial septal defect should have endocarditis prophylaxis before any surgery on an infected or potentially infected area.
3. Over 90% of significant congenital heart lesions can be corrected surgically—some with complete restoration of normal structure and function and some with partial relief of symptoms. If there is any question about diagnosis or treatment of a congenital heart lesion, insist on competent consultation.
4. With better control of prenatal risk factors such as specific virus infections, the occurrence of congenital heart lesions may be expected to drop significantly; lesions like this, however, will always appear, and parents and physicians must always be ready to deal with them.

QUESTIONS FOR PARENTS OF PATIENTS, PATIENTS, AND PHYSICIANS

1. What is the exact anatomic character of this congenital abnormality?
2. Does it represent a shunt between the pulmonary circulation and the general circulation?

3. If it does mean a shunt, how large is the shunt; that is, how much blood would you estimate is flowing through it?
4. If a shunt is present (atrial septal defect, ventricular septal defect, patent ductus arteriosus), is the flow large enough to build up an abnormally high pressure in the blood vessels of the lungs over the years?
5. Should the shunt be closed now, and if not, when should surgery be undertaken?
6. If coarctation is present:
   How severe is the obstruction of the aorta?
   Shouldn't it be repaired surgically?
7. If there is stenosis of the aortic or pulmonic valves:
   Is the stenosis significant?
   What are the prospects for more severe stenosis in later life?
   Is surgery desirable now or is there a possibility that the stenosis will never be a significant problem?
   Isn't endocarditis prophylaxis essential?

17 Medical treatment of heart disease

Most of this book so far has described many things that can go wrong with the heart. This chapter will be a little more cheerful. It will describe the ways the physician can treat the ailing heart. Surgeons can now actually operate on hearts, correcting errors in structure or in some cases undoing the work of various diseases. Surgery is not the only means of helping or curing heart disease. Physicians today have an astonishing armament of drugs and methods. They can make the heart beat faster or slower; can stop abnormal rhythms and restore a normal, efficient beat; can drain excess fluid out of the body through the kidneys, thus taking a great load off the heart; can improve the oxygenation of the tissues; and can do much more. This chapter is not going to try to make an expert therapist out of the nonmedical reader. However, if these methods of treatment are to yield their full benefit, the patient must understand some of the basic ideas involved. Without the patient's intelligent cooperation, the physician is frequently hobbled. In fact, the cardiac patient who cannot or will not follow his physician's instructions may become an invalid needlessly. Worse, he may die, also needlessly.

Until the eighteenth century there wasn't much anyone could do about heart disease. In fact, most of the time nobody knew how to recognize heart disease. Even the brilliant physicians of the Arab world and their equally brilliant successors in the North European Renaissance were in effect as helpful—or as dangerous—as so many blindfolded lunatics with a peddler's pack filled with poisons. Most of the treatment given to cardiac patients throughout the fourteenth, fifteenth, and sixteenth centuries was guaranteed to make the victim much worse; it rarely did any good. By pure, blind coincidence one method of treatment much used by the physicians of that day actually did help cardiac patients; that method was bleeding. Removal of blood by opening a vein was used for almost every disease known to man through the Middle Ages and even through the "Age of Reason." Usually it did a great deal of harm; however, in one case it was very helpful and is still used today. When the cardiac patient is in acute left heart failure, with lungs filled with a great volume of blood, one can relieve the situation almost instantly by withdrawing about a pint of blood through a vein. Without really knowing what they were doing, many physicians of the fifteenth, sixteenth, and seventeenth centuries did help victims of acute left heart failure by opening a vein and letting the patient bleed. It was a case of a stopped clock being right twice a day—they helped the patient purely by accident.

Drug treatment of heart disease really started in the eighteenth century. It is a rather dramatic story. Imagine a man sitting on the stoop of his eighteenth century English home about 1776. He is very sick; he is finding it increasingly difficult to breathe, and he can hardly move about the house without gasping. He has to be propped up on several pillows, and, even so, he must often fight for air. He can tell that his heart is beating rapidly and irregularly, and his ankles are massively swollen. He notices that if he pushes his finger into the tissues of the ankle or shin, he leaves a dent, much as if he pushed his finger into dough. His physician has advised him that he is probably not long for this world and has recommended bringing his will up to date.

At this point an elderly lady comes down the street peddling herb tea. In desperation and on the advice of neighbors the patient begins to drink the lady's herb tea, which she tells him is made from the leaves of the foxglove and is a splendid cure for dropsy, which is certainly what he seems to have. The results are astonishing. In two days he begins to urinate great quantities, and the swelling in the ankles begins to go away. At the same time or even sooner, the heartbeat slows, and the sensation of pounding subsides. He breathes freely and easily, with a vast sense of relief. The improvement is not a passing thing; he finds that he can go about his duties as a country squire as long as he takes the foxglove tea in a measured daily dose. He can walk the estates or even ride to hounds almost as well as in previous years. The improvements last for quite a few years; he learns by experience that if he takes too much of the foxglove tea he becomes nauseated and may feel a sense of extreme weakness and giddiness. With experience, however, he learns to regulate the amount of tea needed for his purposes, and the results continue to astound him and the neighbors.

The disease he actually had, of course, was rheumatic mitral stenosis, which had produced atrial fibrillation with a very rapid ventricular rate. You will remember that this produces a deadly combination of events. First, the narrow opening in the mitral valve causes a great deal of back pressure above the valve in the left atrium and up into the lungs. The lungs, of course, become engorged with blood. Second, the rapid, irregular rhythm of the ventricles makes the heartbeat inefficient, with relatively little blood ejected from the ventricles each minute. Either of these factors by itself can produce heart failure; in combination, the effect is swift and devastating.

What about the foxglove tea? How did it produce its miraculous effect? In the foxglove tea there was an active principle, or chemical, now called digitalis. This is actually not one chemical, but a number of related compounds with similar actions. Digitalis presented the human race with the first really effective agent for the treatment of many forms of heart disease.

TREATMENT OF CONGESTIVE HEART FAILURE
Digitalis

Digitalis compounds have several helpful effects on the heart and circulation. First, digitalis slows conduction of the electric impulse through the atrioventricular node from atria to ventricles. Normally, the cells in the atrioventricular node can pass impulses from top to bottom at a very rapid rate; impulses can pass from the atria to the ventricles as much as 200 times a minute and, rarely, even more often than that. This may not be desirable. If the atria are fibrillating, for example, bombarding the atrioventricular node with over 400 impulses per minute, the ventricles will be driven very rapidly and inefficiently. They never have time to fill between beats, and the output of the heart, that is, the amount of blood pumped per minute, will fall. By giving digitalis, the physician selectively "poisons" the cells in the atrioventricular node so that they will let only a limited number of beats through per minute. In this way the physician can slow the rate of the wildly beating ventricles down to a normal level, providing more efficient ejection of blood with each beat. Again, think of the analogy of squeezing a bulb syringe, using slow, steady squeezes, allowing the bulb to fill completely before compressing it. By slowing the ventricular rate to a normal level, this is exactly the effect one produces on the heart.

Digitalis, in other words, produces a kind of block, or delay, in the cells of the atrioventricular node. This delay may be very helpful if too many impulses are trying to pass through these cells. By regulating the rate of passage through these cells, the physician regulates the rate of the heart.

The patient will feel the effect of improved ventricular pumping almost at once; the increased blood pumped per minute is frequently lifesaving in itself.

Second, digitalis has a direct effect on the heart muscle. By some means not yet well understood, digitalis increases the efficiency of contraction in the heart muscle, and the ventricles pump more blood per stroke and per minute. When a person with a failing heart is given digitalis, the amount of blood pumped out of the left ventricle frequently rises as much as 30% with each beat. Thus even if our imaginary eighteenth century patient had a normal heart rhythm to begin with, the digitalis would still have been helpful in improving ventricular performance up to a level that would maintain his life.

Finally, digitalis acts as a diuretic. This means that the drug causes an increased passage of fluid out of the body through the kidneys as urine. This diuretic effect of digitalis is really a secondary result of its effect on the heart. By improving the amount of blood pumped by the heart, digitalis also increases the circulation of blood through the kidneys and hence the amount of water removed from the blood as urine.

It is now easy to understand why the country squire of 1776 felt so much better a week after taking the foxglove tea. The basic cause of the heart disease was still present. The chances were that he would die of it; however, the heart had been strengthened and made to beat efficiently, and the load of extra fluid had been drained from the body so that the heart and circulation could cope with the diseased valve and still sustain life. During the next two centuries an enormous amount of study was devoted to this drug, and many preparations are now available for physicians. The old foxglove tea was widely inaccurate in dosage. The man who took a teaspoon of it might be taking a quarter of what he needed or might be taking ten times the maximum safe dose. Toxic reactions were very common and, in fact, dangerous. Today the physician can control the level and the action of digitalis with a very high degree of accuracy; the drug can be given by mouth or by vein. There is much controversy about just what kinds of heart disease should be treated with digitalis, and there are legitimate differences of opinion among experts. However, there is universal agreement that it is useful if not essential in a great variety of cardiac irregularities and that it is often needed in heart failure of almost any cause.

Toxic effects

By its very nature, digitalis can be a very dangerous drug; too much digitalis can kill. The drug must be given under close medical supervision, and even when the patient has been maintained in good control, frequent rechecks are needed. Certain dangerous irregularities of heart rhythm may be caused by digitalis; the block produced in the atrioventricular node may become so severe that the heart may slow to a dangerous level. Side effects include nausea, vomiting, and distortion of vision. The patient taking digitalis should probably have the pulse and other cardiac findings checked once a month; failure to have adequate supervision can result in serious and sometimes fatal complications.

Morphine

The narcotic drug morphine is astonishingly useful in certain types of heart disease. This is especially true in acute left heart failure and in treatment of myocardial infarction when the patient suffers much pain. The great Soma Weiss, physician at the Peter Bent Brigham Hospital in Boston, used to quiz applicants for internship. One of his favorite questions was, "What is the most useful single drug in the treatment of heart disease?" The answer Dr. Weiss wanted was not, as one might suppose, digitalis or quinidine but rather morphine.

In the chapter on left heart failure you will remember certain abnormal reflexes were described. These reflexes go into action when the lungs are engorged with blood and produce rapid, gasping, inefficient breathing. This abnormal breathing makes the situation a great deal worse than it need be. The effect is heightened by the apprehension or even frank terror that often grips these patients. A hypodermic dose of morphine blocks the abnormal reflexes to the lungs and calms the patient; the effect is sometimes astonishing.

I have seen patients in acute left heart failure, gasping, blue, obviously desperately ill, who were given an injection of morphine at home while waiting for the ambulance. By the time the ambulance had arrived at the hospital, their condition had improved by at least half. Their color was better, their breathing was easier, and they were obviously out of the touch-and-go stage of the disease. The action of morphine in blocking the abnormal nerve reflexes to the lungs and in promoting more efficient breathing is enough to tip the scales back in the patient's favor.

When occlusion of a coronary artery produces a myocardial infarct, pain and fright combine in a dangerous way. Pain itself may throw a patient into shock; the shock, or drop in blood pressure, then produces a less efficient circulation of blood through the coronary arteries, and a vicious cycle has been started. Again, administration of enough morphine to stop the pain, calm the patient, and prevent the descent into shock is frequently lifesaving.

One need hardly point out the dangers in the indiscriminate use of morphine. This is a habit-forming drug, and it is all too easy for a patient to become an addict. However, with intelligent medical supervision, morphine may well mean the difference between success and failure in acute cardiac emergencies. In recent years other synthetic pain-relieving drugs have been developed that approximate the action of morphine, but all share with morphine the frightening possibility of drug addiction.

Oxygen

Remember the heart is basically an oxygen pump. When the heart fails for any reason, the oxygen supply of all the tissues, including the heart muscle, drops to a critical level. By giving the patient pure oxygen to breathe, one raises the oxygen level in the cells of the body and takes a great work load off the straining heart. Oxygen will practically always be used in the acute stage of heart failure and will be used in many cases of acute coronary insufficiency or occlusion. Even oxygen, however, is not harmless. In some cases it must be used with great caution. In some types of chronic cor pulmonale (Chapter 7) the indiscriminate use of oxygen may be dangerous. In some cases oxygen can produce death through a kind of coma. You may begin to tire of this warning, but it still holds true; oxygen, like other cardiac therapeutic agents, must be used only under medical supervision.

Diuresis

The patient in heart failure has too much blood circulating in his body. Most of the time he also has too much fluid in his tissues. One could simplify this by saying that the patient in heart failure has too much water in his body; one would be approximately correct.

Removal of this excess fluid through the kidneys is called **diuresis,** and it is one of the most useful procedures available to the physician treating heart disease. Various drugs will cause the kidneys to pass out, or excrete, large quantities of water as urine. Certain types of diet will do the same thing.

The key to control of edema fluid in the tissues is the mineral called sodium. Everyone has eaten large quantities of sodium combined with chlorine to form sodium chloride, or table salt. Sodium is present in the body in many forms and in many combinations. In edema fluid the sodium concentration is extremely strong. This fluid is actually a kind of "brine." If the physician can make the sodium move out through the kidneys, the water in which the sodium is dissolved will "follow the sodium out" as urine. To do this, it is usually necessary to cut down on the amount of sodium the patient takes in. Since the most common source of sodium is table salt, this will usually be cut down in cardiac diets when it is necessary to pull edema fluid out of the tissues. One should remember that this is really the only time that restriction of sodium is helpful in heart disease as such; the number of fairy tales about the effect of salt on the heart are astounding. They are all based on misinterpretation of this one elementary fact.

A number of drugs are now available which will cause excess fluid to leave the tissues by way of the kidneys. These drugs have somewhat different modes of action, but generally speaking, they promote passage of sodium out of the body in the urine. The sodium "takes water with it" and the excess fluid drains out of the body. The effect of this kind of diuretic is sometimes dramatic, with a loss of many pounds of weight in twenty-four hours and an equally dramatic relief of shortness of breath and other distress associated with congestive heart failure. In many cases of mild congestive heart failure diuresis is all that is needed. Simple removal of the extra fluid load from the body makes it possible for the patient to breathe and function normally.

You may wonder how long this kind of artifical drainage of edema fluid can be kept up. The answer is that it can be maintained in many cases for a number of years. I have seen cardiac patients continue to enjoy a normal or nearly normal existence, thanks to diuretic therapy, for fifteen or twenty years. At the end of that time they had lived out a reasonable life expectancy for anybody.

Again, a caution! It is very easy when draining edema fluid through the kidneys to upset the chemical balance of the minerals in the body. For example, certain diuretic drugs will cause the potassium to fall to a dangerously low level in the tissues and in the blood. The same is true of the sodium and the chloride, which are all vital elements in the body's chemistry. Careful medical supervision and repeated checks of these levels in the blood are essential if the diuresis is to succeed and if the patient is to avoid dangerous complications.

Vasodilators

In the past ten years a new approach to treating congestive heart failure has been perfected; it involves the use of drugs that dilate the arteries so that it is easier for the heart to pump blood out into the vessels of the body. By "opening up" the arteries into which the blood is being pumped, the resistance to flow is lowered and a considerable load is taken off the left ventricle. Some of these drugs also dilate the veins, thus holding a certain amount of fluid out in the tissues, away from the heart and lungs, and reducing the amount of work the heart has to do.

Nitroprusside

This is a drug which can be given only by vein, but it is very quickly effective. It dilates, or "opens up," both the arteries and the veins and hence reduces the amount of work the heart has to do in pumping blood out into the vessels of the body. It also reduces the amount of blood returning to the heart from the veins, thus lowering the total volume that has to be pumped. This drug has to be used with very careful control, of course, because it is possible to drop the blood pressure too far or to reduce the circulating volume too much. Properly used, this drug is often lifesaving; it is also very useful for the acute treatment of severe elevations of blood pressure.

Prazosin

Prazosin is a drug that can be taken in tablet form, and it has much the same action as nitroprusside—that is, it dilates both arteries and veins, thereby "unloading" the heart.

Hydralazine

Hydralazine works only on the arteries; it is a very efficient dilator of the small arteries and thus decreases the work of the left ventricle very quickly. It has an unfortunate side effect of increasing heart rate, but this can be countered by the use of other drugs. It also has a long-term complication of producing a reaction in the connective tissues in the body called "lupus erythematosus." Anyone taking hydralazine for long periods should have blood tests for this particular complication.

Nitroglycerin and isosorbide

Nitroglycerin and isosorbide are both described in the section on treatment of coronary artery disease, but, in brief, both drugs can be used to help relieve left heart failure, again by simply dilating the veins and "trapping" a certain amount of fluid out in the tissues of the body, thereby reducing the load to be pumped by the heart.

Rotating tourniquets

Although the utility of tourniquets has been questioned by some investigators lately, there seems little serious doubt that properly applied tourniquets high on the arms and legs can relieve many cases of acute heart failure by trapping blood in the extremities. Tourniquets should be applied only by nurses, physicians, or individuals with advanced medical training, since there is the hazard of cutting off the blood flow to the limbs. The tourniquets are applied as high as possible on both arms and both thighs and are tightened so that the veins are shut off but the arteries are not; the physician or nurse will always take the pulse at both wrists and in both feet very carefully to ensure that the arterial blood flow is normal. By this treatment a great deal of blood is pumped out to the limbs, which does not return through the partly stopped up veins, and again the heart is "unloaded."

CONTROL OF ARRHYTHMIAS
Digitalis

The effect of digitalis in slowing the ventricular rate in the presence of atrial fibrillation has already been described. Digitalis is also useful for paroxysmal tachycardia arising in the upper part of the heart, that is, in the atria or in the atrioventricular nodal region. It is effective in atrial flutter, again by slowing the rate of conduction from the rapidly fluttering atria to the ventricles and protecting the ventricles from the excessively rapid beating of the atria. Digitalis may also convert a flutter or fibrillation to a normal rhythm indirectly by improving cardiac output, dropping the pressure in the atria, and improving the flow of blood through the coronary arteries as a result of the improved pumping action of the left ventricle. CAUTION: Digitalis can cause as many arrhythmias as it cures; many patients take digitalis along with diuretic agents, and this combination, unless controlled, can be dangerous. Certain diuretic agents cause excessive amounts of potassium to flow out of the body in the urine; the combination of the low blood level of potassium with digitalis can produce several forms of rapid, dangerous heart rhythms. Anyone taking digitalis and a diuretic should always take an agent which replaces potassium in the body, and the level of potassium in the blood should be checked. Digitalis can also produce any form of paroxysmal tachycardia, atrial, nodal, or ventricular, and is a common cause of ventricular ectopic beats.

Quinidine

Quinine, the extract of the bark of the cinchona tree of South America, has been put to a tremendous number of uses. A few decades ago every person with an obscure fever was diagnosed as having malaria and dosed heavily with quinine. More recently it has been used to give a bitter flavor to tonics for no very good reason. However, quinine or its chemical cousin quinidine is an extremely useful and very powerful cardiac medication. Quinidine is used only to regulate disorders of the heart rhythm. It does not have any of the other actions of digitalis, although some of its effects on the heart rhythm are very like those of digitalis. One of the chief effects of quinidine is the suppression of abnormal rhythms in any of the chambers of the heart. For example, quinidine will often stop ectopic beats whether they arise in the atria or in the ventricles. It will control many cases of paroxysmal tachycardia, regardless of the part of the heart in which the tachycardia originates. Quinidine will often stop a fibrillation in the atria and start a normal rhythm in these chambers. Used in conjunction with digitalis, quinidine will often control atrial flutter and bring about a normal beat.

Quinidine does not have the helpful effect of digitalis on the heart muscle nor does it have any diuretic action in draining edema fluid out of the tissues. Its only effect is on abnormal rhythms in the heart.

Toxicity

Quinidine slows conduction from atria to ventricles, primarily in the bundle-branch system and to a lesser extent in the atrioventricular node. Quinidine can produce any type of heart block, and toxic levels can produce death through cardiac standstill. These side effects are not described to frighten the patient out of using a very useful drug; they are simply another reason for close medical supervision when a powerful agent like quinidine is being taken. I have had patients take quinidine for ten or fifteen years without harmful effects. On the other hand, I have seen people in real trouble within a few weeks when they have not been properly supervised. Don't wander off on a vacation or an extended trip overseas with a pocketful of digitalis or quinidine without making arrangements for medical supervision.

Procainamide

Procainamide is a drug chemically related to the procaine that the dentist puts in your jaw to make it numb; it has been very useful in controlling certain abnormal rhythms, particular ventricular tachycardia or ventricular ectopic beating. It is also effective in certain atrial arrhythmias, that is, fibrillation or flutter, but less so than quinidine. Procainamide can be given by vein under close supervision, or it can be taken in tablet form. Until recently procainamide had to be taken every three hours to be effective; a longer acting preparation is now on the market which may solve this particular problem, since it has to be taken only two or three times a day.

Toxicity

Procainamide, like hydralazine, can produce a "lupus" reaction in the connective tissues of the body; anyone who has been taking procainamide for more than two or three months should be checked for this phenomenon.

Disopyramide (Norpace)

Disopyramide is a drug rather like quinidine, used almost exclusively for treating ventricular ectopic firing. It is chiefly prescribed for control of ventricular tachycardia or ventricular ectopic beats.

Toxicity

Disopyramide can depress left ventricular function and actually produce congestive heart failure, particularly if the ventricle was damaged to start with. Its use must be monitored very carefully, especially in patients with any evidence of impaired left ventricular function.

Diphenylhydantoin (Dilantin)

This drug has been used for years to control epilepsy. It is very useful in one specific kind of arrhythmia—ventricular ectopic firing produced by digitalis toxicity. In this situation it is often lifesaving.

Lidocaine

This chemical cousin of procainamide and procaine has proved a boon in the treatment of ventricular arrhythmias, that is, ventricular tachycardia or ventricular premature beats. The drug is so safe and so effective that it is given routinely in many coronary care units to any patient who has suffered a myocardial infarct. It has the great advantages of low toxicity and quick excretion; after the medicine is stopped it leaves the body in a very short time. It can be given only by vein and should be used only in a setting such as a coronary care unit, where intensive monitoring is routine.

Verapamil

This is one of a new class of drugs only recently available to American physicians, although they have been used abroad for many years. These drugs act by blocking the flow of calcium across the cellular membrane and hence slowing conduction through parts of the heart. Verapamil slows conduction through the atrioventricular node and in this way has some of the effects of digitalis. It is chiefly useful in patients with atrial fibrillation when the ventricular response cannot be controlled with digitalis preparations; verapamil alone or in combination with digitalis is very useful in this specific setting.

Propranolol

The "beta-blocking" drugs have several uses; in the arrhythmias propranolol is specifically useful in combination with digitalis to slow conduction from atria to ventricles when the atria are going too fast. Thus with atrial flutter or fibrillation, when digitalis alone does not slow the heart rate sufficiently, sometimes the addition of propranolol will bring the rate into reasonable control.

Toxicity

The beta-blocking drugs have some important toxic effects. They depress left ventricular function so that the left ventricle pumps less efficiently, and in cases where the left ventricle was damaged or inefficient to start with, this can produce actual congestive heart failure. In addition, by their nerve-blocking action they can make asthma a great deal worse; no one who has a history of asthma should take these drugs.

Electroversion

By delivering an electric shock precisely timed with the patient's own heart cycle, it is possible to end certain arrhythmias. Atrial fibrillation, atrial flutter, and any type of paroxysmal tachycardia may respond to cardioversion. If a rapid, abnormal rhythm is reducing the efficiency of the heart to a dangerous level, sometimes electroversion is the quickest and safest approach to control a dangerously rapid rhythm of the heart.

TREATMENT OF CORONARY ARTERY INSUFFICIENCY

Unfortunately there are no medicines that will "unharden" a coronary artery or cause the atheroma to disappear. The drugs available are used primarily to reduce the oxygen requirements of the heart muscle and hence help the heart to pump an adequate amount of blood even though the blood flow to some parts of the heart muscle is diminished.

Nitroglycerin

In large quantities nitroglycerin makes an excellent explosive; it is frequently used to open safes under illegal conditions. In tiny quantities nitroglycerin is one of the best agents in the treatment of coronary heart disease.

During the siege of Paris in the Franco-Prussian War, an intelligent French physician noticed a curious reaction among the workmen on the barricades. These men were handling cases of dynamite, inhaling dust and fumes in great quantities. They began complaining of a peculiar reaction in which their faces were flushed and their heads seemed to pound and throb.

The physician realized that this was apparently a reaction of the blood vessels in the head and various parts of the body to inhaling the fumes of nitroglycerin. He noticed that the faces of these men turned a bright red color and that the small blood vessels seemed to be hugely enlarged, or dilated. Their hearts had a rapid pounding action, and the whole effect was quite unpleasant.

He described this phenomenon, labeling it the **nitritoid effect.** Simple reasoning led to the use of this same phenomenon medically in diseases in which blood vessels were constricted, leading to inadequate blood flow to tissues. The most obvious disease of this class, of course, is angina pectoris, and nitroglycerin happened to be of tremendous benefit in this field. In Chapter 6 on coronary disease the action of nitroglycerin and its chemical cousin isosorbide is described.

Drug companies have spent prodigious amounts of time and money trying to develop a long-acting coronary dilator. In other words, they have been trying to find a drug that would cause the coronary arteries to dilate and stay dilated for hours or days. These attempts have not been successful to date, and it is likely that the benefits patients describe after taking these long-acting coronary dilators is simply the age-old effect of power of suggestion. Most cardiologists regard these presumed long-acting drugs with a very skeptical eye.

Repeated use of nitroglycerin does not lessen its effectiveness. The drug is not habit forming and has no significant side effects. The patient can take nitroglycerin or its chemical cousin amyl nitrite for years with benefit and without harmful toxic effects. Just how the drug works is still the subject of some debate; it seems clear, however, that the chief effect of the drug is dropping the resistance to the outflow of blood from the left ventricle into the arteries and, more importantly, dilating the veins so that a large quantity of blood is "trapped" in them. This sudden "unloading" of the left ventricle drops the oxygen requirements of the heart muscle. The blood flow that had previously been inadequate is now sufficient for the reduced needs of the heart muscle cells and the anginal episode is halted. There is also some evidence that nitroglycerin may dilate coronary arteries, although this is probably a minor part of its action. Nitroglycerin can also be applied to the skin in a form of paste. Surprisingly, the medication is absorbed into the bloodstream and is very effective. Nitroglycerin paste applied to any area of skin, twice a day, has emerged as a very useful long-term medication for the treatment of severe angina pectoris.

The modern use of nitroglycerin emphasizes prophylaxis; in other words, a patient with angina pectoris should take nitroglycerin before performing any level of physical activity that usually brings on discomfort. Thus before walking to the store, climbing a flight of stairs, or performing some manual labor, the patient with angina pectoris should place a tablet of nitroglycerin under the tongue, let it take effect, then go ahead with the activity. This prophylactic use of nitroglycerin greatly enhances the total effect of this drug.

Isosorbide taken under the tongue in the same manner as nitroglycerin appears to have an effect that lasts about three or four times as long. When swallowed in large doses of 10 milligrams three or four times a day, the drug has a continuous twenty-four–hour effect in dilating the veins and "unloading" the left ventricular myocardium. That is an important part of the treatment of chronic coronary artery disease.

Beta blockade

Beta blockade is a tremendous advance in the treatment of coronary artery disease. A drug called propanolol has been discovered and brought into general use within the past ten years. This amazing chemical has the effect of blocking certain sympathetic nerve fibers so that they cannot exert their usual effect on a number of organs in the body, including the heart. This beta-blocking effect means that the heart will beat more slowly and somewhat less strongly. At first this might seem a contradiction: why should one give a drug that would actually "weaken" the heart? The answer is that the oxygen needs of the heart muscle vary with the rate of the heartbeat and the strength of the contraction. Any engine running faster or more powerfully will always need more fuel. If the engine can do the same job more slowly or with less powerful thrust, less fuel will be demanded. The fuel here, of course, is oxygen supplied by the heart muscle through diseased coronary arteries. Beta-blocking drugs enable the heart to carry out its required pumping action with less consumption of fuel.

Beta blockade, curiously, reduces coronary blood flow somewhat, but the important point is that it reduces the *requirements* of the heart muscle more than it reduces the flow, so the net effect is a plus. The heart muscle receives more blood relative to its reduced needs, and the patient functions more efficiently and frequently without anginal pain.

Beta blockade has been a godsend for patients with angina pectoris. Many of them have been able to resume normal productive lives due to the amazingly selective action of the beta-blocking drugs. One reason for the increased efficiency of the heart with lower "fuel" consumption is that the body extracts more oxygen from each liter of blood so that same amount of oxygen will be taken into the body at the cost of less mechanical energy exerted by the heart.

Toxicity

Beta-blocking drugs, like many potent medications, are two-edged swords: the very "slowing down" effects on the heart that the drug is expected to produce may also lead to trouble if the patient is not carefully observed. If the heartbeat is weakened too much, or if the rate is too slow, the patient can go into congestive heart failure or can begin to faint because of inadequate delivery of blood to the brain. Patients with asthma should *never* take beta-blocking drugs; the peculiar nerve-blocking effect of these drugs can cause very dangerous constriction of the air passages. If a patient is aware of asthma, the physician should be alerted to this fact. Beta-blocking drugs obviously should be administered only be physicians who are thoroughly familiar with their advantages, disadvantages, and toxicity and who are sufficiently skilled in cardiac diagnosis to detect the earliest signs of inadequate cardiac performance.

Nifedipine

Nifedipine, like verapamil, is a drug that works by blocking the movement of calcium into the cells. It is odd that although nifedipine and verapamil are very similar, they have quite different effects in the heart. The nidefipine works to block spasm, or temporary constriction, of coronary arteries. New investigation suggests that this kind of temporary constriction plays a very important role in many kinds of coronary artery disease; spasm together with coronary atheromatous degeneration is thought to play a role in the production of myocardial infarcts. In a patient with Prinzmetal angina, that is, angina not related to exertion, nifedipine can have a very dramatic effect, since this form of angina is often caused only by spasm of the vessels in the absence of any organic disease. When patients with angina pectoris have not responded to the usual management with nitroglycerin, isosorbide, or beta-blockers, the addition of nifedipine sometimes relieves symptoms very dramatically and permits resumption of a nearly normal existence.

Toxicity

Nifedipine depresses left ventricular function about as much as the beta-blocking drugs do and can actually produce congestive heart failure. If a patient taking nifedipine notices that shortness of breath is becoming more severe or more frequent, the physician should be alerted at once. Nifedipine will usually be prescribed with considerable caution if the physician is aware of depressed left ventricular function.

• • •

You should conclude this chapter by remembering a couple of points: First, an amazing number of cardiac therapeutic agents are now in hand to correct the heart rate and rhythm, clear the body of edema fluid, restore proper oxygenation to the tissues, and, to some estent, offset the effects of disease of the coronary arteries. Patients can be helped, even in the face of severe heart disease, to live a normal, useful life.

Second, it must be written in letters of flame that every one of these agents is powerful and potentially dangerous, if not lethal. They should be used only under expert medical direction with continuing supervision. I have seen many tragedies follow the careless use of these drugs; overdosage or underdosage may be equally dangerous. One of the really frightening abuses of cardiac therapeutic drugs takes place when the urge to be helpful overwhelms some cardiac patient to the point of telling a friend to try some of his medication "because it helped me!" On any label of cardiac medication the patient should imagine a picture of a very sharp two-edged sword. Medication is a weapon that can help or can hurt; it can cure or it can kill. Handle with care!

18 Cardiac catheterization

Catheterization of the heart for diagnostic purposes has been described in Chapter 6 on coronary artery disease and on valvular disease. Cardiac catheterization is a common diagnostic tool; it is performed thousands of times every day in the United States.

The patient who is told that a heart catheterization is necessary always has questions about the procedure.

What is actually going to happen? Is it going to hurt? Is it dangerous? What information is the cardiologist going to find that couldn't be found by a stethoscope, an electrocardiogram, or some other means?

Catheterization of the heart had an interesting beginning; in the 1920s a rash young German researcher named Forseman decided to see if injecting cardiac drugs directly into the heart would make them more effective. Since all veins drain into the right heart, Forseman simply introduced a long, thin, flexible, hollow tube (called a catheter) into a vein in his arm and then actually threaded it up the vein, through the shoulder, into the chest, through the great veins and into the right side of his heart. He then went down to the x-ray department and had an x-ray picture taken, which showed that, indeed, the catheter had advanced into what was apparently the right ventricle.

Forseman was extremely lucky that he didn't die of his procedure, considering the state of technology at that time. His original idea about injecting drugs directly into the heart was not correct, but the technique itself opened the door on a whole new world of possibilities in cardiac diagnosis.

The technique is best described by explaining some of its specific applications.

CATHETERIZATION OF THE RIGHT HEART

This is a relatively simple, safe procedure. A catheter (Fig. 18-1) is filled with saline solution and connected to a reservoir of fluid so that it can be continuously flushed out. It is introduced to a vein in the arm, in the neck, or in the groin and simply threaded up through the veins into the right side of the heart. The catheter will pass through the right atrium, the right ventricle, and finally out into the pulmonary artery. The physician will generally use a fluoroscope to tell by x-ray visualization exactly where the catheter is throughout the procedure.

Findings recorded in right heart catheterization
Pressure

By attaching a pressure recorder to the outside end of the catheter, the cardiologist can record the pressure in the right atrium, the right ventricle, and the pulmonary artery. The pressure waves are different in each area, and the physician can often tell where the catheter is simply by looking at the pressure tracing, without even using the fluoroscope.

Right heart catheterization

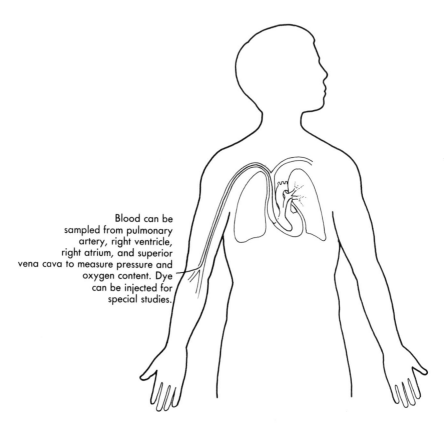

Blood can be
sampled from pulmonary
artery, right ventricle,
right atrium, and superior
vena cava to measure pressure and
oxygen content. Dye
can be injected for
special studies.

Fig. 18-1. Diagram of right-heart catheterization.

Diagnosis of pulmonic stenosis

If there is narrowing at the pulmonic valve, the pressure in the right ventricle, "upstream" from the narrowing, will be abnormally high, while the pressure in the pulmonary artery, "downstream" from the valve, will be abnormally low. By measuring the difference in pressure above and below the narrowed valve, the physician can calculate how severe the narrowing is, that is, how small the hole is in the pulmonic valve. This will be a key measurement in deciding whether surgery is necessary.

The drop in pressure across an abnormally narrowed valve from the high-pressure area above to the low-pressure area below is called the "pressure gradient." It is an extremely important measurement in assessing the need for valve surgery.

A remarkably simple, ingenious form of right heart catheter has been designed by Dr. Swan and Dr. Ganz; it is often used in a coronary care unit to decide if the left heart is failing or not. Remember that if the left heart is failing, an abnormally high pressure will "back up" progressively through the left atrium, the pulmonary veins, and finally the pulmonary arteries. Measuring the pressure in the pulmonary arteries and getting an idea of the state of function of the left ventricle sometimes is a matter of life and death and has to be done very quickly. The Swan-Ganz catheter has at its tip a tiny inflatable balloon, which acts rather like a sail; the catheter can be "floated" through the right heart, into the pulmonary artery, and all the way out to the smallest vessels, where the catheter finally wedges itself in place. The measurements taken with this type of catheter tell with great accuracy whether the left ventricle is failing; it is in common use in every well-equipped coronary care unit.

Oxygen measurements

If there is a hole in the septum between the atria or the ventricles, the arterial blood, rich in oxygen, will move through the hole into the right side of the heart, where the blood, being venous, is normally low in oxygen. During right heart catheterization, if the cardiologist suspects such a hole, or septal defect, measurements of oxygen levels of the blood will often give the needed information. If the blood sample in the right atrium, for example, has an oxygen content of about 70%, and the blood sample from the right ventricle suddenly shows an oxygen content of over 80%, it is clear that there must have been a "leak" of oxygen-rich blood from the left ventricle into the right ventricle to produce this rise. In other words, there must be a ventricular septal defect. By noticing how much the oxygen content of the blood increases, the cardiologist can calculate the amount of blood flowing from the left side of the heart into the right side through the septal defect. This kind of calculation gives a rough but adequate idea of the size of the defect itself, at least in functional terms; it is often the crucial measurement in deciding whether surgery is necessary.

Angiography

If structural abnormalities are suspected, such as the more complicated kinds of congenital heart disease, the cardiologist may inject dye into the right ventricle and take successive cineangiograms, or x-ray movies, as the dye is pumped out of the heart.

●   ●   ●

The chief and commonest reasons for catheterizing the right side of the heart will be (1) disease of the pulmonic or tricuspid valves, (2) congenital heart disease, (3) Swan-Ganz catheterization to estimate left ventricular function.

LEFT HEART CATHETERIZATION

To catheterize the left side of the heart it is necessary to put the catheter into an artery, usually in the arm or the groin, and thread it "upstream" against the flow of blood into the aorta, through the aortic valve, and into the left heart itself. This is a much more complicated procedure than right heart catheterization,

Left heart catheterization

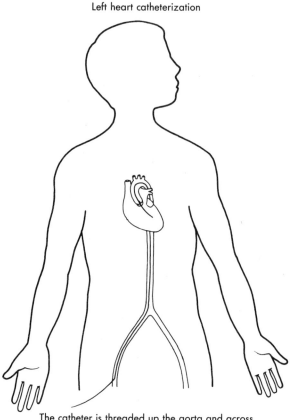

The catheter is threaded up the aorta and across the aortic valve into the left ventricle. This permits measurement of pressures in the aorta and left ventricle. Dye can be injected to measure left ventricular function and to detect "leaking" in the mitral valve.

Fig. 18-2. Diagram of left-heart catheterization.

and it is about ten times as risky. Since the catheter is moving against the flow of blood rather than with it, fluoroscopic guidance is always necessary to see the exact location of the catheter tip; it cannot simply be "floated" into position as is often the case with a right heart catheter (Fig. 18-2).

Uses of left heart catheterization
Aortic or mitral stenosis

Stenosis, or leakage, of the aortic or mitral valves can be assessed by catheterization. When stenosis is suspected, the gradient, that is, the pressure above and below the valve, will be the key measurement.

In aortic stenosis this is relatively simple to obtain; with the catheter in the left ventricle, pressure is recorded, and then the catheter is withdrawn through the aortic valve to the aorta, where the pressure is again recorded. The drop in systolic pressure between the ventricle and aorta is the pressure gradient across the narrowed valve, and as a general rule, the higher the gradient, the narrower the opening in the valve.

Mitral stenosis measurements are a little more complicated; at the end of diastolic filling of the ventricle, when the mitral valve is wide open, there should be no pressure gradient between the left atrium and the left ventricle. When the mitral valve is narrowed, or stenotic, however, the blood above the valve in the left atrium has not finished running into the left ventricle by the end of diastolic relaxation, simply because the hole through which it runs is too narrow. Therefore at the end of filling, when there should be no gradient at all, there will still be a higher pressure in the left atrium than in the left ventricle. Again, a gradient exists, and the severity of this gradient tells the physician how severe the narrowing is in the mitral valve.

Regurgitation, or leaking, of valves is harder to measure and must be done by indirect means, including injecting dye downstream from the valve and seeing how much of the dye leaks back through the valve. Pressure measurements are also helpful, although indirect calculations have to be used.

Left ventricular function

For many years cardiologists and researchers have worked on the problem of measuring left ventricular function; the conclusion is that the *ejection fraction* is the most accurate measurement of left ventricular function. The term "ejection fraction" simply means the percentage of blood in the ventricle at the end of diastole that is ejected during systole. Normally about 60% of the total volume of the blood is ejected with each systole; if the ventricle is failing, a smaller percentage is ejected, and in a diseased ventricle the percentage may fall to as low as 30% or 20%. This ejection fraction is best measured by injecting dye into the left ventricle and then measuring successive x-ray picture frames very carefully as the dye is ejected in the next systole. By doing this in two dimensions the cardiologist can make a very accurate measurement of the ejection fraction. This measurement will often be the deciding factor when cardiac surgery is proposed, since a patient with a very low ejection fraction faces a very high risk when undergoing cardiac surgery. Information about the ejection fraction, that is, the function of the left ventricle, is sometimes the most important data obtained by catheterizing the left side of the heart.

Congenital heart lesions

When congenital heart lesions involve the left side of the heart, catheterization of the aorta, left ventricle, and even occasionally the left atrium will be essential to define the precise relationships of the abnormal structures in the heart and to permit corrective surgery. Cineangiography and measurement of pressures and of blood oxygen levels will all be brought into play in many of these complex abnormalities.

CORONARY CINEANGIOGRAPHY

The astonishing technique of coronary cineangiography developed by Dr. Mason Sones represents one of the great advances of twentieth century cardiology. By using properly shaped catheters, the cardiologist can actually thread the catheter into the openings of the left and right coronary arteries, inject dye under pressure into these structures, and produce remarkably clear pictures of the arteries and their small branches (Fig. 18-4). Coronary arteriography is not necessary in every case of coronary artery disease, since the necessary information can often be obtained by electrocardiography, treadmill testing, or even by a carefully elicited history of symptoms. The precise indications that justify coronary arteriography are listed in Chapter 6. These are listed in some detail because coronary

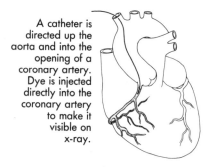

A catheter is directed up the aorta and into the opening of a coronary artery. Dye is injected directly into the coronary artery to make it visible on x-ray.

Fig. 18-3. Coronary arteriography.

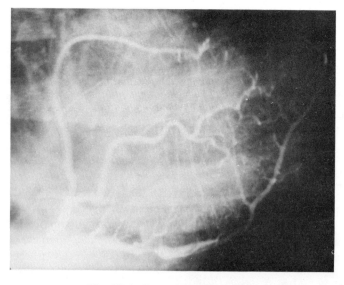

Fig. 18-4. Coronary angiography.

arteriography has probably been overutilized and even abused more than any technique in modern cardiology. Before a patient submits to the procedure, it should be very clear that there is ample justification. The questions listed in Chapter 6 should be posed and answered, and if there is the slightest doubt, consultation by a disinterested, uninvolved cardiologist should be invoked.

Coronary arteriography carries a certain risk: in a well-run catheterization laboratory this will be in the range of about 0.1%, meaning that one person out of every thousand will die of the procedure. There is also a risk of stroke, myocardial infarction, and clotting in the artery used for the catheterization.

Coronary arteriography should be carried out only be a highly skilled cardiologist who has had specific training in the technique in the course of an approved fellowship. The catheterizing cardiologist and the supporting team should carry out several procedures a week to maintain skills and should be able to respond rapidly and effectively to the emergencies that will predictably arise. The "occasional" cardiac catheterizer who carries out a few procedures a year probably represents an unacceptable risk to the patient; it takes practice and constant rehearsal of techniques to perform with an adequate degree of safety.

WHAT IT'S LIKE TO HAVE A HEART CATHETERIZATION

Cardiac catheterization should never be painful; the cardiologist will use a local anesthetic before the catheter is threaded into a vessel, and about the only sensation the patient will ever feel is a burning flush when the dye is actually injected inside the heart or in the great vessels. During coronary arteriography the patient may feel pain like the pain of angina pectoris or myocardial infarction. This can often be relieved by injecting nitroglycerin directly into the coronary artery through the catheter. During catheterization of the left heart or the coronary arteries abnormalities of heart rhythm are common; an alert catheterization team can usually correct these within seconds.

A final word about cardiac catheterization in general: A cardiologist should be able to make 95% of all cardiac diagnoses by what are called "noninvasive" measures. The history of the illness, the physical examination, the electrocardiogram, the x-ray examination, the echocardiograms, and at times nuclear medicine studies should give almost all the information needed. Cardiac catheterization is a "court of last resort" to make precise, quantitative determinations that are necessary for cardiac surgery or at times to clear up the remaining 5% of diagnostic information that cannot be obtained by other means.

Cardiac catheterization should never be the first step in cardiac diagnosis; it should usually be the last.

19 Cardiac surgery: how it is done and what it is like

Surgery on the heart is commonplace today; before World War II it was considered a fantasy. In a number of sections of this book cardiac surgery has been described as a treatment for congenital abnormalities, valvular heart disease, and coronary artery disease. Cardiac patients should have a general idea of how this is all done, what the risks are, and what the benefits may be.

Until the late 1940s surgery on the living heart seemed impossible; after all, it was an organ which was beating continuously and filled with blood, and any incision into it would result in massive hemorrhage and death.

Cardiac surgery really became possible with the invention of the heart-lung machine. This remarkable piece of equipment performs the functions of both the heart and the lungs, that is, it oxygenates the blood and clears it of carbon dioxide, and then pumps it on through the vessels of the body with sufficient force to make it circulate adequately.

The way the heart-lung machine works is shown diagrammatically in Fig. 19-1. Briefly, tubes are placed in the two great veins returning blood to the heart; all the blood is then short-circuited into the heart-lung machine, and after the blood has been properly oxygenated it is returned to the aorta and thence to the arteries of the body. Thus the heart and lungs are completely taken out of the circulatory system during the operation.

It would be very difficult to operate on a heart if it were beating continuously, so the heartbeat is stopped, commonly by simply cooling the heart down with a controlled atmosphere of slush, or sometimes by using chemicals to stop the heartbeat.

The surgeon now has a still, blood-free organ on which to operate; correction of abnormalities can be carried out very deliberately and precisely.

WHAT THE SURGEON ACTUALLY DOES
Congenital heart disease
Defects outside of the heart

Patent ductus arteriosus. The simplest operation for congenital abnormality is the repair of a patent ductus arteriosus. This canal between the aorta and pulmonary artery actually lies outside the heart, and the surgeon does not even have to use the artificial heart pump to correct it. The chest is opened, both ends of the short, wide, abnormal vessel are clamped, the ends are cut and sutured, and the operation is over.

Coarctation of the aorta. Like patent ductus arteriosus, coarctation of the aorta can be corrected without invading the heart and hence without using the

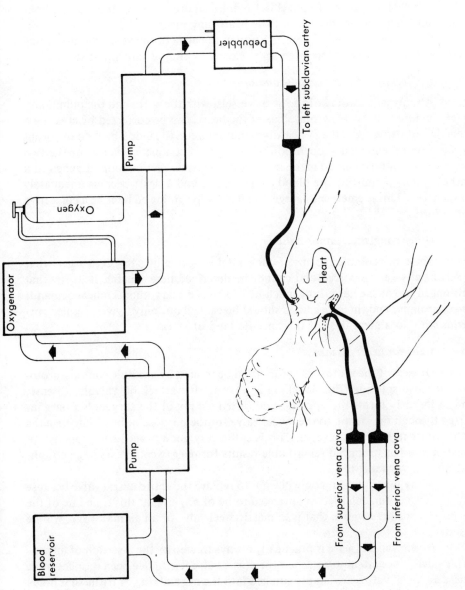

Fig. 19-1. The heart-lung machine.

heart pump. The aorta is clamped above and below the narrow place, the abnormal tissue is cut away, and a graft is stitched in.

Defects within the heart

Most other types of congenital repair require work on the inside of the heart and hence will involve use of the heart-lung machine.

Septal defects. Septal defects between the atria or the ventricles are closed by a patch if the hole is too large to be closed by simply suturing it shut.

Defects of the great vessels' anatomy

Abnormal anatomy of the great vessels, with the aorta and the pulmonary artery coming out of the wrong sides of the heart, can be corrected by creating a "baffle" of tissue from the pericardium that redirects the blood back to the proper side. As an emergency operation when there is complete reversal of the two great vessels, a hole can be made in the atrial septum by a balloon attached to a catheter, thus permitting the blood to recirculate and at least become adequately oxygenated. This is emergency surgery and is always followed later be a corrective procedure.

Other congenital abnormalities

The more complex forms of congenital abnormalities involve surgery that is technically very involved and cannot be described here. Suffice it to say that prolonged use of the heart-lung machine will be necessary, the technical demands are enormous, and the procedures should be carried out only by very skilled surgeons who do a great deal of this specific kind of work.

Valvular heart disease

Disease of the mitral valve can often be treated by a simple commissurotomy, or valve splitting (Fig. 19-2). This was the first attack on valvular disease, and in its early forms the operation consisted simply of the surgeon's finger inserted through the atrium to the mitral valve for the purpose of breaking open the adhesions and freeing the valve. This is still a very good procedure, properly applied, and it has produced remarkable results for over twenty years in a substantial number of patients.

Many times the surgeon will want to replace the entire mitral valve because the leaflets are too calcified or shriveled to be of any use; at this time one of the forms of prosthetic valve, that is, a plastic-steel valve or an animal valve, will be inserted.

Aortic valve disease is practically always treated by the insertion of an artificial valve, since attempts to repair the aortic valve itself have been unsuccessful. These artificial valves are simply stitched into the normal ring of tissue that holds the natural valve. To do this, of course, the patient's own valve must be carefully cut away.

Disease of the pulmonic valve—practically always congenital—is treated by simply cutting the valve open; very rarely is a prosthetic valve used in the pulmonic position (Fig. 19-3).

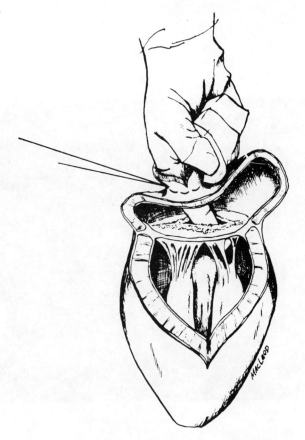

Fig. 19-2. Mitral commissurotomy.

The same is true of the tricuspid valve; I have been involved in only one case which required a prosthetic tricuspid valve; when correction is needed it can usually be accomplished by surgical repair of the patient's own valve tissue (Fig. 19-4).

Coronary bypass surgery

As described in Chapter 6, on coronary artery disease, this is a "detouring," or bypassing procedure; veins from the patient's legs or, more rarely, arms are attached to the aorta a short distance past the heart and stitched into the patient's coronary arteries somewhere beyond the point of obstruction. It is common to put in three, four, or even five grafts; this is sound surgical procedure because a number of these grafts will predictably stop up in the first six months after surgery, and thus the more grafts there are, the better chance the patient has of having some improvement from the procedure.

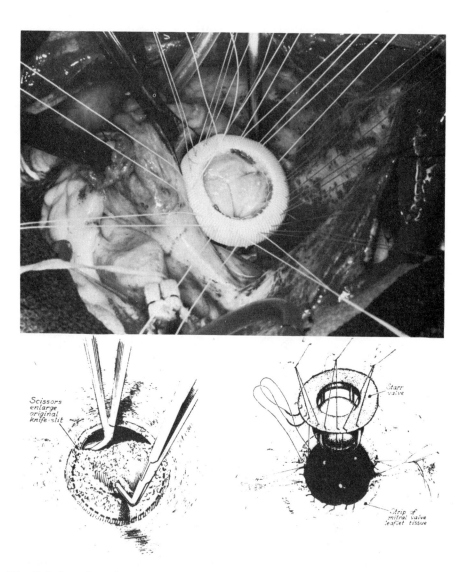

Fig. 19-3. Insertion of prosthetic valve. (Illustration courtesy of Dr. Jack Copeland, University of Arizona Medical Center.)

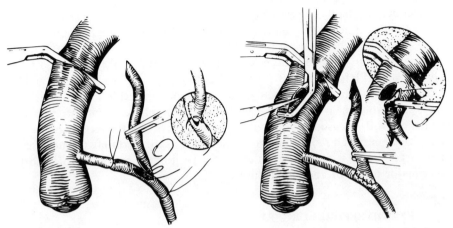

Fig. 19-4. Coronary bypass surgery. (Courtesy Dr. Jack Copeland, University of Arizona Medical Center.)

RISKS OF SURGERY

What are the risks of cardiac surgery? Of course, no general statement can be made. The risk of closure of a patent ductus arteriosus or of correction of a coarctation of the aorta is extremely small—certainly less than 1%. The risk involved in the more complicated forms of congenital heart disease is directly proportional to the complexity of the congenital abnormality: the more repairs that have to be made, naturally, the higher the risk, other things being equal.

Most of the common types of congenital abnormality of the heart can be corrected with no greater risk than that involved, for example, in surgery for stomach ulcers or gallstones.

Valvular surgery

The risk of valve surgery depends on the stage of the disease: if the heart has been allowed to deteriorate too much because of an abnormal valve, the risk of surgery is proportionately high. On the other hand, if the time for surgical repair is well chosen, at the exact point when the patient's symptoms demand surgery yet cardiac structure and function have not deteriorated past "the point of no return," the risk is very reasonable and again is probably on the order of 1% to 2%—no more than the risk involved in any major abdominal surgery, for example. If the patient has complicating disease such as emphysema or if the left ventricle has deteriorated severely, the risk will be proportionately higher.

Coronary artery disease

The risks of surgery for coronary artery disease have been summarized in Chapter 6. To state them briefly, the risk of operating on the left-main vessel is quite high in comparison with surgery of the other coronary arteries—left-main vessel surgery probably carries a mortality of about 10%, although this figure will vary a great deal depending on the skill and experience of the surgeon.

Surgery on the other coronary arteries generally carries a risk that is directly proportional to the degree of impairment of left ventricular function, just as in valve disease. If left ventricular function has seriously declined (reflected in a low ejection fraction), the risk will be significantly higher than if left ventricular function is somewhere near normal. To give an overall figure, coronary artery disease in a patient with a reasonably functioning ventricle, except for surgery of the left-main vessel, carries a risk of not more than 2%, again, certainly no more severe than surgery for a ruptured peptic ulcer, for peritonitis, or for any of a host of other major forms of abdominal surgery.

PERIOD BEFORE SURGERY

The most important point to be made about the period before surgery is that it almost never has to be hurried. With three rare exceptions, there is for practical purposes no such thing as emergency cardiac surgery. The patient and the patient's family should never be stampeded into surgery on the pretext that it is a matter of life and death that the surgery be carried out in the next few hours. In all the ordinary forms of coronary disease that present a reasonable basis for surgery—crescendo angina, uncontrollable angina pectoris, or angina pectoris after a myocardial infarct associated with left-main disease or three-vessel disease, clinical studies all over the United States and the world have shown that the patient always benefits by a "cooling off" and stabilizing period prior to surgery. There is always time to relieve the acute symptoms and balance the supply-and-demand ratio of blood in the heart muscle before the patient is subjected to surgery.

EMERGENCY SURGERY

There are a few instances in which emergency surgery is necessary.

Complete transposition of the great vessels

When a child is born with the aorta coming out of the right ventricle and the pulmonary artery coming out of the left ventricle without any other communication between the pulmonary circulation and the general circulation, emergency surgery is needed. A catheter must be passed through the normal small hole between the atria and by balloon inflation a larger hole must be created, permitting mixing of pulmonary and arterial blood and thereby saving the infant's life. This is called a Rashkind procedure, and its prompt performance is quite literally a matter of life and death.

Complications of myocardial infarction

Two rare complications of myocardial infarction may be helped by surgery. They are rupture of the attachments of the mitral valve so that the valve swings free, leaking an enormous amount of blood up into the left atrium, thereby producing abrupt and basically untreatable congestive heart failure, and rupture of the tissue in the interventricular septum because it has been damaged by a myocardial infarct, with creation of a septal defect between left ventricle and right ventricle. These patients will become critically ill very quickly and will usually die. Surgery immediately after myocardial infarct is very hazardous, but when either of these two complications appear, the cardiologist and the cardiac surgeon may have no choice but to recommend rapid lifesaving surgery.

In every other manifestation of coronary disease, however, the patient and the patient's family, on being told that surgery is an emergency, should always demand consultation. It never really is.

COMMUNICATION, COMMUNICATION, COMMUNICATION

The thoughtful, competent cardiologist and cardiac surgeon will insist on thorough and repeated explanations of the kind of surgery that should be performed, the need for its performance, and the risks associated with it to the patient and to the close family. If patients do not receive this kind of information, they should be ready to demand it; if there is anything about the procedure or the disease that necessitates it that the patient and his close family do not understand, they should ask repeatedly for information until the whole process is crystal clear in everyone's mind. The patient should never be bashful about asking for information; sometimes physicians act harrassed and hurried, but the patient shouldn't be put off by the appearance of bruskness or by the use of involved technical terms. After all, it's the patient's heart and the patient's life that are at stake; if anyone doubts the need for surgery or the precise character of the procedure, consultation should be demanded.

As a physician who has practiced for forty years in a number of settings, I always encourage patients to request consultation and will frequently request it myself, even though the patient doesn't. The physician who is reluctant to ask for a consultant's opinion is quite often a physician who is personally insecure or sometimes simply suffers from a personality disorder that produces anger or suspicion when consultation is requested. The hallmark of the wise and confident physician is the frequent use of consultants and the prompt and courteous cooperation with any request for consultation from the patient or the patient's family.

FURTHER NOTE TO PATIENTS: When you ask for a consultant, be sure you get someone who is competent! Patients are very often fond of physicians because of a pleasant personality or a deep and genuine concern that the physician manifests toward their various minor aches and pains. This doesn't mean that said physician is competent to judge highly technical points involving cardiac diagnosis or surgery. It usually doesn't cost any more to get an opinion from the most highly qualified physician in your region. Check with the local medical school, hospital staffs, county medical society, or the offices of the specialty groups such as the American College of Cardiology or the American College of Physicians for lists of names of physicians with adequate training and established competence in a particular field.

The patient's own emotional state is enormously important in cardiac surgery or, indeed, in any cardiac crisis, and it is important that the patient be totally satisfied as to the accuracy of diagnosis and the adequacy of what is being done. This can make physical differences, such as lowering of epinephrine (natural adrenalin) levels in the blood, which may rise with anxiety. The patient's emotional state may really spell the difference between success and failure in cardiac procedures.

In summary, before submitting to cardiac surgery, remember that there is never any rush; ask questions until everybody is perfectly clear and satisfied; feel free to ask for competent consultation. Clearing the air of doubt and uncertainty, fear and suspicion will help everyone concerned, including the attending physician.

20 Special diagnostic techniques: echocardiography and radioisotope studies

ECHOCARDIOGRAPHY

One of the reasons the Allies won both world wars was that their navies learned to detect enemy submarines underwater. They did this by sending out sound waves through an area of the ocean and listening for the echoes when these same sound waves "bounced back" from various objects beneath the surface.

This same technique, called sonography, is now used to map the contours of organs inside the human body. Ultrashort sound waves are sent through the part of the body being studied, and by adjusting the depth of the echo-detecting equipment, specific organs and tissues can be outlined with remarkable accuracy.

Echocardiographic recordings of the heart make it possible to "take a picture" that shows the size of the chambers, the thickness of the ventricular walls, the motion of the valves, and the size of the valve openings.

Echocardiograms can be recorded by a "single-view" technique called the "M-mode," or by computer-assisted multiple recordings that permit what amounts to a three-dimensional visualization of all the major structures in the heart (Fig. 20-1).

Echocardiography has found some clear-cut uses in the diagnosis of cardiac disease.

Chamber size

It is possible to measure the diameter of several of the chambers in the heart, as well as the thickness of their walls, very accurately. Since the only other way to do this would be to catheterize the heart and inject dye directly into the chambers, the usefulness of a simple, safe technique like echocardiography is obvious. By knowing chamber size, the cardiologist is often able to deduce the severity of certain valve lesions. Progressive enlargement of the left ventricle past a certain point, for example, in the presence of aortic regurgitation, may be the most reliable single piece of information that indicates that the time for surgery has arrived.

A large left atrium and right ventricle with a small left ventricle would fit the pattern of severe mitral stenosis, while progressive enlargement of the left atrium and left ventricle may present important clues about the need for surgery when the patient suffers from mitral regurgitation.

Valve structure (Fig. 20-2)

The mitral valve can be well-visualized most of the time by echocardiography. The diagnosis of mitral stenosis specifically has been greatly simplified by echocardiographic techniques. Visualization of the aortic valve is possible with

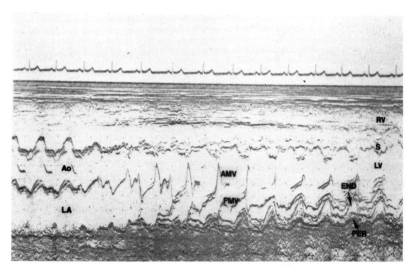

Fig. 20-1. Normal echocardiogram. (Courtesy Gordon Ewy, M.D., University of Arizona Medical Center.)

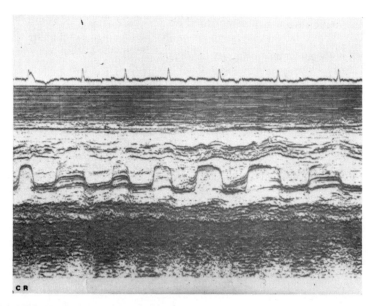

Fig. 20-2. Echocardiogram of severe mitral stenosis. (Courtesy Gordon Ewy, M.D., University of Arizona Medical Center.)

the "sector scanner" or the "3-D" type of echocardiogram; visualization of the aortic valve with the "single-view," or M-mode technique has been less helpful. The pulmonic and mitral valves can also be visualized in many patients, but it is much more difficult technically to do so.

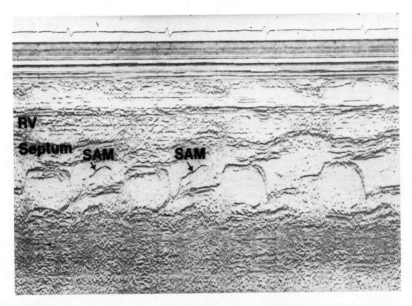

Fig. 20-3. Echocardiogram of idiopathic hypertrophic subaortic stenosis. (Courtesy Gordon Ewy, M.D., University of Arizona Medical Center.)

Deformities of muscular structure

Since the wall thickness can be measured throughout the various parts of the heart cycle, that is, throughout systole and diastole, echocardiograms can give information about the presence of thin, scarred areas, or abnormally thickened areas. One disease with the impressive name of **idiopathic hypertrophic subaortic stenosis** (Fig. 20-3) can be specifically diagnosed with very satisfying accuracy by echocardiographic means. In this disease the septal wall is thickened and the cells themselves are disorganized because of an inherited disorder of growth. This thickening makes an hourglass-shaped obstruction in the middle of the left ventricle that delays the ejection of blood from the chamber. Echocardiography is the definitive method of diagnosis of this particular disorder.

Congenital heart disease

The more sophisticated types of echocardiography have opened a whole new world of possibilities in the diagnosis of congenital heart disease. The subject is too technical to review here, but it is safe to say that any pediatric cardiologist should have very thorough grounding in the technique. The findings are sometimes so accurate that a definitive diagnosis can be established on the basis of the echocardiogram alone.

Coronary artery disease

In a startling advance it has been shown that echocardiography permits visualization of the first part of the left-main coronary artery. Since disease of the left-main coronary artery is the most dangerous form of coronary disease, the possibility of visualizing this structure without the difficulties and hazards of catheterization is very exciting. At this time the technique would have to be classified as experimental, but the rapid advances in this and related fields make it likely that noninvasive visualization of all the structures of the heart, including the coronary arteries, will be possible before another decade has passed.

RADIOISOTOPE DIAGNOSIS

The technique of using radioactive "tracer" elements in the diagnosis of heart disease is really in its infancy; it is not possible yet to say just how useful it will be. Radioactive elements can be used in the diagnosis of heart disease in two different ways.

Differentiation of "live" from "dead" tissue in the heart muscle

When heart muscle cells die, usually because their blood supply has been cut off, they are replaced by scar tissue, an inert white mass. The cells in this scar tissue are, of course, completely different from normal, healthy, functioning heart muscle cells.

Certain radioactive elements, when injected, will be "picked up" selectively only by healthy heart muscle cells with a normal blood supply flowing to each of them. These elements will not be picked up by dead scar tissue. By injecting such an element and recording the radiation from the heart, it is therefore possible to outline areas of scarring in the heart wall. Thus if there were a suspicion of previous myocardial infarct that could not be resolved by electrocardiographic or other means, the demonstration of an area where no radiation could be recorded and hence presumably there were no living cells might settle the question.

When the blood supply to cells is cut down drastically, as during angina pectoris, radioactive elements will not concentrate as well as they do in areas with a normal circulation. It was hoped that by exercising patients on a treadmill to the point of electrocardiographic change or anginal pain and then injecting radioactive material, it would be possible to pick up the difference in concentration of radiation between the cells with inadequate blood flow and those with normal blood flow. This technique has presented many problems, and although initial results were encouraging, it is clear that it is not yet a completely accurate method (Fig. 20-4, *A* and *B*).

Measurements of wall motion and chamber size

Other isotopes can be injected which will give different levels of radiation from the pool of blood inside the chambers of the heart and the cardiac tissues themselves. Using very sophisticated computer techniques and measuring the differences in radiation throughout the heart cycle, it is possible to project a color image of the beating heart on a screen. Different levels of radiation are represented by different colors, and with computer addition techniques a dynamic image of the beating heart can be visualized.

The chief use of this kind of study so far has been the determination of ejection fraction of the left ventricle. Since this is the most important and the

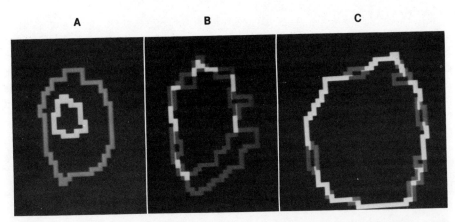

Fig. 20-4. Outline of the heart in systole and diastole using radioisotope techniques. The outside line represents the maximum diameter of the heart in diastole; the inside line represents the smallest set of diameters in systole. The calculation of the difference between the two permits analysis of an ejection fraction or ventricular efficiency. **A,** Normal ejection fraction. Notice the large difference between the outline in diastole and systole. **B,** Poor ejection fraction. Notice that the heart does not move in as much as in **A;** that is, there is less difference between diastole and systole, meaning a poorer ejection fraction. **C,** Very severe heart disease with extremely poor ventricular function; notice that there is almost no difference between diastolic and systolic outlines.

most sensitive measurement of ventricular function, this application alone has brought radioisotope techniques into the field of practical diagnostic cardiology.

Research possibilities

By using computer subtraction techniques, it is possible to visualize certain blood vessels based on the difference in concentration of an isotope inside and outside of the vessel. This may even be possible for the coronary arteries someday, and of course this opens the most promising of all possibilities. If it were possible to visualize the coronary arteries by the simple injection of a radioisotope into a vein, cardiology would be revolutionized. The diagnosis of coronary artery lesions would be made incredibly simple, and a great many catheterization laboratories would go out of business. This, of course, is only in the realm of research, but it's promising.

Nature of radioisotopes

The radioisotopes used in "nuclear" cardiology are very short lived and they do not subject the body to any significant amount of radiation. The instruments used to detect them are so sensitive that very tiny doses can be used, and elements are chosen with a half-life of a few hours, meaning that the radiation is gone in a very short time. The amount of radiation involved in the performance of most of these tests is less than the patient would undergo having a simple x-ray examination of the chest.

CAVEAT

• Nuclear medicine is, to a great extent, experimental, and the yield so far has been limited. Before a patient spends a great deal of money on nuclear cardiac tests, there should be considerable frank discussion about what information is being sought and why. At this time the determination of ejection fraction is probably the major practical application of the method, and the times when a cardiologist will need to know precisely what an ejection fraction is in quantitative terms will really be very few.

21   The heart patient and work

Heart disease is almost never a reason to stop human activity. Except for the desperately ill patient requiring oxygen therapy, almost everyone who suffers from heart disease can and should do some kind of work. The question is, "What kind of work and how much?" There is nothing worse than the vegetable existence some cardiac patients embrace as soon as they discover they have heart disease. The human animal needs to be challenged to put forth some kind of productive effort. In the absence of challenge the individual fails physically and mentally.

Coronary heart disease, in terms of work, can be separated from almost all other forms. The work approach differs in the coronary patient as compared to the patient with valvular heart disease, congenital heart disease, or hypertensive heart disease. Since coronary heart disease is one of the most common kinds of cardiac abnormality, this will be considered first.

CORONARY HEART DISEASE

People who suffer some clinical manifestation of coronary disease—myocardial infarction or angina pectoris—often suppose that they have been placed on a shelf to spend the rest of their lives sipping beef tea and smiling at comforters with a wan, sweet smile. This is pernicious nonsense. Two presidents of the United States have suffered myocardial infarctions and have gone on to run for presidency and subsequently serve in this post, which can hardly be called restful. Any number of hard-working, creative individuals in the arts, the sciences, and the business world have lived through one and sometimes more coronary attacks and have gone on to fulfill happy, useful lives. Myocardial infarction or angina pectoris is never to be regarded as an excuse for taking the veil and retiring from active life.

The habits of life that predispose to coronary disease have been described in Chapter 14. Assume that the patient has gone into all these personality problems at length with his physician. There still remains the question of what he can do. *Physical exercise, properly controlled, is of great benefit to most patients who have coronary artery disease.* Remember that collateral circulation, that is, cross-connection between the coronary arteries, is not very good. Suitable amounts of exercise taken at frequent intervals under proper supervision are probably the strongest stimulant to growth of better collateral circulation in the heart muscle. If the patient's employment can provide this kind of steady, controlled physical exertion within the limits of what is safe for him, the employment will not only be harmless but will also probably be helpful.

Mental tension and psychic exhaustion are known to be important factors in coronary artery disease. The hard-driving executive who rushes to make deadlines, harasses his subordinates, and worries about his superiors is actually doing everything he can in mental terms to bring on a coronary attack. If coronary artery disease appears, the patient must be ready to abjure the silly, compulsive, scrambling activity that characterizes much of our business and professional world. The patient must be prepared to work at a reasonable rate with adequate periods of rest and interludes of relaxation. He must be ready to ignore the neurotic individuals around him who try to unload their tensions. He must set himself larger, longer range goals than the simple-minded acquisition of wealth that

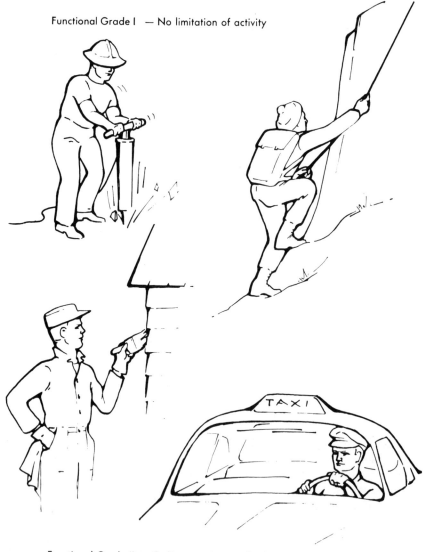

Functional Grade I — No limitation of activity

Functional Grade II — Ordinary activity well tolerated, strenuous activity producing distress

Fig. 21-1. Functional capacity in heart disease.

is the curse of so much of our culture. He must think in terms of years rather than days. He must carry on his mental work at a steady, reasonable rate in an atmosphere as free of tension and needless crises as can be achieved. He must be prepared to go to great lengths and possibly to make some sacrifices to attain this atmosphere.

With these rules in mind, one can approach the problem of what the patient can do in physical terms. This brings up the work classification study, which has been a tremendous boon in the rehabilitation of cardiac patients. In a work classification study the patient performs physical exercise under controlled conditions with observation of heart rate, blood pressure, and electrocardiogram during and after exercise. Every conceivable kind of employment has been studied in terms of physical energy required for it (Fig. 21-1).

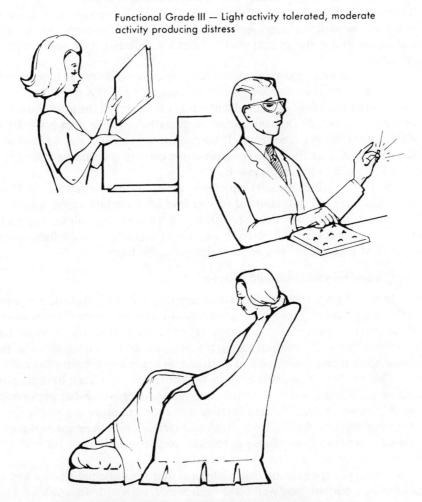

Functional Grade III — Light activity tolerated, moderate activity producing distress

Functional Grade IV — Symptoms present even at rest

Fig. 21-1, cont'd. Functional capacity in heart disease.

Waiters, advertising agency executives, cowboys, lumbermen, carpenters, plumbers, soldiers, and sailors have all been studied very carefully by experts in the field of work classification. One can predict with great accuracy the number of calories per hour the patient is burning up as he carries out his normal daily activity. It is not hard to put the patient who has suffered some kind of coronary artery episode through a comparable level of exercise in the laboratory, observing his heart carefully all the while. One of the most useful instruments for controlled exercise is the treadmill. The patient simply walks on a large treadmill that runs at a controlled speed. It is tilted at a known angle so that the patient may walk on the flat, up a gentle hill, or up a very steep mountain. By controlling the grade tilt on the treadmill and the speed of the machine, the examiner can produce almost any energy output he wishes. With monitoring equipment, the electrocardiogram is recorded continuously during work performance. The pulse rate and blood pressure are checked at frequent intervals. The bicycle ergometer, a stationary bicycle that the patient pumps against an electric load, is another useful way of providing controlled energy output. The heart is monitored in the same way as on the treadmill.

If the pulse rate speeds abnormally or remains rapid for too long a time, if the blood pressure rises above the level of normal, or if the electrocardiogram shows the kind of change associated with acute blood lack in the heart muscle, the observer may conclude that the patient is doing more work than his heart can safely maintain. On the other hand, if the patient can carry on a given level of exertion without any of these abnormalities, one can assume that he can carry on this kind of work in his employment.

Work classification units have been set up in many parts of the United States. They have put thousands of former invalids back into useful, productive work. Often the man who has been sitting in an armchair thinking himself a hopeless invalid proves to be perfectly capable of carrying on some light or moderate kind of physical activity with no danger to his heart.

Cardiac rehabilitation and exercise

In recent years there has been an attempt to utilize controlled, progressive exercise as a means of rehabilitating victims of coronary artery disease. In most of these rehabilitation units the patient is tested on a treadmill to assess basic work tolerance and is then put through a program of increasing physical exertion—usually running—with careful electrocardiographic monitoring throughout.

This has been a laudable project, but the results have been to some extent disappointing. Controlled progressive exercise *does* improve cardiac performance in many patients: it *does* increase exercise tolerance and make it possible for patients to expand their capabilities in work and recreation. It *does not* prolong life. The basic coronary artery disease pursues its course regardless of the prescribed exercise unless other risk factors are modified.

The secondary gain of better physical and mental conditioning and improved mental outlook may well make such a program worth undertaking. However, anybody with significant coronary artery disease would probably do well to discuss pros and cons with the attending cardiologist.

OTHER TYPES OF HEART DISEASE

Valvular heart disease and congenital heart disease are another matter. In these two diseases work classification is extremely important, and it is carried out just as in the case of the coronary patient. There is an important difference, however; when a diseased valve throws a load on the heart or when an inborn abnormality of the heart overloads the circulation, physical exercise is not much help in improving the patient's functional state. In fact, it may be very dangerous.

If the heart is pumping against a narrowed aortic valve or a leaking mitral valve, the extra load of physical exercise does not improve the patient at all. In cases like these the object of work classification is to find a means of livelihood that the patient can carry on within the limits of cardiac function. Most of the skilled types of work are well within the capabilities of the majority of people suffering from valvular or congenital heart disease. A man who could not work as a farmer, oil-rig worker, or longshoreman could work for years as an expert in carburetor repair, a gunsmith, a jeweler, or a barber. Vocational rehabilitation units set up in many parts of the country reeducate patients with physical handicaps for new ocupations. This kind of retraining has prevented thousands of men in the prime of their life from becoming wards of the state. It is one of the most useful functions of our government at any level.

The man with serious valvular heart disease may have to change his kind of work, but he can practically always be trained to do something that will support him and his family without aggravating his heart disease. Again, very careful work classification study is vital if the patient is to learn what kind of work he can safely carry out.

To sum up, the patient suffering from any type of heart disease should consult at length with his physician, and, if it seems advisable, careful work evaluation studies should be carried out. The patient will then have a good idea of his capabilities and his limits. He can seek gainful employment of a suitable kind and can work productively without fear.

22 What to do about a heart attack

Half of all deaths are caused by disease of the heart and blood vessels. The chances are good, therefore, that you will be on hand when someone actually has a heart attack. It is a common occurrence.

If the heart attack strikes on the golf course, on a fishing stream, during a backpack trip, on a ski slope, or any place far from medical aid, what can you do?

There are only a few things that the nonmedical person can do for the victim of a heart attack. These few things, however, may be very important. There are also some things that you should not do.

A heart attack will be one of two disorders: (1) acute left heart failure or (2) some type of coronary artery syndrome.

ACUTE LEFT HEART FAILURE

The symptom of acute left heart failure will be shortness of breath. The victim will not necessarily say "I am very short of breath"; apprehension, anxiety, and fear of sudden death may all be the first symptoms actually described, but rapid panting and sometimes agonized breathing will be obvious. The color of the lips and earlobes may be blue, and there is frequently a white frothy material about the lips. The patient will refuse to lie down flat and will only feel comfortable sitting up; the patient, in fact, will usually resist any attempt to force him to a lying position. The patient is fighting for breath because the lungs are engorged with blood, trapped in back of a failing left heart. (Review Chapter 3 and be sure you understand the mechanism of acute left heart failure.)

Rotating tourniquets

In an area remote from medical aid there is really only one immediate maneuver that helps the patient in acute left heart failure. This maneuver should only be carried out by someone with advanced first aid training, preferably at a paramedic level. This procedure is called **rotating tourniquets.**

Place tourniquets around the arms and legs as high as they can be placed on each member. These tourniquets can be strips of cloth, heavy rubber bands, neckties, handerchiefs, or anything that can be knotted or twisted. *While applying the tourniquets, feel for a pulse in the member the tourniquet is being applied to; do not turn the tourniquet so tight that it turns off the pulse in the wrist or in the feet.* The point of applying these tourniquets is to stop up the veins but *not* to stop up the flow of blood out to the limbs through the arteries. Otherwise, they would serve no purpose and would endanger the patient's circulation to the extremities. Therefore tighten tourniquets enough to stop up the veins and halt the return of blood to the heart, but do not tighten the tourniquets enough to turn off the arterial pulse. Always check for arterial pulses in the limb to which the tourniquet is being applied. Send for help. In about five or ten minutes the patient will usually begin to breathe more easily. When this happens, loosen one of the tourniquets, leaving the other three tight. Every fifteen minutes retighten the loose tourniquet and loosen another one—in other words, rotate the tourniquets.

You can keep up this rotation of tourniquets for several hours while you wait for any needed help to arrive. If you are really in the wilderness, days from help, you can start to release the tourniquets one at a time after a couple of hours if the breathing seems easier. The tourniquets can always be reapplied if needed.

Don't try to make the patient walk about. *Don't* throw cold water on his face. *Don't* try to give him artificial respiration. *Don't* try to make him eat or drink anything—he won't want to, and he shouldn't.

CORONARY HEART ATTACKS

These will be either angina pectoris, myocardial ischemia, or a myocardial infarct. The symptom will be pain or some other acute discomfort, usually in the front of the chest. It may go up the sides of the neck toward the jaws. It often goes down the arms, particularly the left arm. Sometimes the pain will be in the very upper part of the abdomen, just at the lower end of the breastbone. The victim may think that he has *acute indigestion,* and he will almost always be frightened or apprehensive.

Angina pectoris

If the patient is a known sufferer from angina pectoris, help him to take his nitroglycerin, amyl nitrite, or other quick-acting coronary dilator. Help him find a place to rest, and watch him while the pain goes away. If it is a typical attack and he is used to them, he will be able to resume activity when the pain has disappeared.

Myocardial ischemia and myocardial infarction

The pain will not go away, even with rest or with nitroglycerin. The discomfort persists, and the patient is usually very apprehensive. You can do these things:

1. Put the patient at rest in a chair, couch, or bed. Sometimes he will want to move about and walk around in a frightened, agitated manner. Don't let him do it. Make him be quiet.
2. Relieve the pain. Aspirin, whiskey, or any of the common pain-relieving agents available are all useful. Alcohol is good because it relieves pain and calms the frightened, agitated patient.
3. Send for help. Even if this means waiting for horses, jeeps, helicopter, or some other means of travel out of rugged country, don't move the patient until help arrives.

Don't move the patient about or let him move himself about; keep him quiet. *Don't* force him to eat; foods and liquids should be given in very small quantities as he desires them. *Don't* apply artificial respiration or give stimulants such as caffeine.

"STOPPAGE" OF THE HEART

Acute left heart failure or coronary disease of any kind may cause the heart to stop pumping blood. This may happen in one of two ways: the ventricles may simply stop beating and hang motionless (ventricular standstill, Chapter 17, Fig. 17-4, *B*) or the ventricles may go into a feeble twitching motion, which cannot pump any blood (ventricular fibrillation, Chapter 17, Fig. 17-4, *A*).

In either case the patient will fall as though shot. He will be motionless, and he will not breathe. He is not yet dead, and he does not really have to die in many cases. Surprisingly often his life can be saved if there is someone nearby who knows what to do.

Remember, the patient is not breathing and his heart is not beating. In three or four minutes the cells of the brain will begin to die for lack of oxygen. What is to be done must be done at once.

Following are the steps in cardiopulmonary resuscitation:

1. Establish unresponsiveness. Tap the patient, gently shake the patient, or shout loudly to see if the patient will rouse.
2. Summon help.
3. Get the patient in position for resuscitation (straighten the legs, get the patient flat on the back).

These first three steps should not take more than five or ten seconds.

4. Establish presence of cardiopulmonary arrest: Check for breathlessness; look for evidence of breathing motions in the chest or upper abdomen or for movement of air through the nose or mouth. Feel for a pulse in the wrist or in the neck.
5. While actually carrying out these observations, prepare the airway by tipping the head back and pulling the lower jaw up or forward. At the same time observe the mouth to see if there is fluid, vomit, or other material in it. If such material is present, turn the head to one side and clean the mouth thoroughly with a handkerchief, shirttail, or any material available before beginning resuscitation.
6. Begin mouth-to-mouth breathing by pinching the nose shut, placing your mouth around the victim's mouth tightly, and blowing air in, watching to see that the chest actually expands. Ventilate the patient with four breaths of fresh air, making sure, of course, to inhale fresh air between each forced breath into the patient.
7. If at the end of this time the patient is pulseless and unconscious, begin closed chest massage. Kneeling at the side of the patient, place the heel of one hand on the sternum. Place the other hand on top of it and make sure that the fingers themselves are not actually touching the chest. Begin to depress the sternum at least 1½ to 2 inches and then release the pressure completely rather quickly so that the heart will refill, but do not remove the hands from the sternum.

8. Keep up a ratio of fifteen chest compressions for two breaths until the patient revives or until additional help arrives.
9. If a second rescuer becomes available who is skilled in cardiopulmonary resuscitation, have one rescuer perform the compressions and the other the breathing with a ratio of five compressions to one breath. Periodically recheck for a pulse or for signs of spontaneous breathing, at which time the effort, of course, can be stopped.

This is a brief outline of cardiopulmonary resuscitation. The American Heart Association and various hospital staffs give much more detailed instruction in how to carry this out, and it is safe to say that almost anyone would benefit from taking these courses. They are available in every community in the United States. Certainly close relatives of patients with heart disease should be thoroughly familiar with cardiopulmonary resuscitation. In Seattle, a city which has led the world in organizing this kind of emergency resuscitation, it was found that cardiopulmonary resuscitation by bystanders who happen to have training gave far and away the best results in terms of lives saved, since they began their measures immediately without waiting for ambulances or paramedics.

Read these basic steps over in any case and have them so well memorized that you'll carry them out systematically, no matter how many terrified amateurs are giving the wrong advice or getting in the way. Sometimes life will return in an astonishingly short time. I have seen a heart begin to beat and a patient begin to breathe within ten seconds. It is certainly tragic to think of a human life wasted for the want of such a simple lifesaving procedure.

If the accident happens in civilized surroundings, keep going until medical aid arrives, even if this takes an hour. Many patients have lived after two hours of closed chest massage and mouth-to-mouth breathing. In the wilderness, far from any possible help, one should think of an hour as the minimum time to continue the effort. In the absence of skilled medical help don't assume the patient is dead or beyond hope. However, at the end of an hour if the patient shows obvious signs of death, it is probably time to give up.

When the patient is actually dead beyond reviving, the pupils of the eyes will become very large. The lips, nail beds, and ears will all be distinctly blue. The patient will be making no attempt to breathe on his own, and there will be no detectable pulse.

If you have never seen anyone die, stoppage of the heart is likely to produce panic. *Don't run for help. Don't go rummaging about in people's bags looking for aspirin or other pills. Don't run for a glass of cold water or a telephone. In other words, don't do any of the hundred and one foolish things people usually do in this kind of emergency.*

To reiterate, the simple measures outlined here applied by nonmedical personnel have probably saved more lives annually than half the technologic wizardry available to the medical profession. Every competent adult should be thoroughly trained in cardiopulmonary resuscitation; the measures outlined should be a drill that is gone through swiftly, systematically, and without deviation in the event of cardiopulmonary arrest. The potential benefits are enormous.

Low-cholesterol diet (approximately 150 milligrams) for type IIa hyperlipoproteinemia*

When cholesterol in a diet is being controlled, there is a decrease in saturated fats and an increase in unsaturated fats. The diet is the same as the Type IIa hyperlipoproteinemia diet. This diet provides an adequate amount of the nutrients as indicated by the RDA.

Foods permitted	Foods to avoid
Milk group	
Three cups of skim milk, powdered skim milk, evaporated skim milk, or low-fat buttermilk; skim-milk yogurt	Whole milk in any form, condensed milk, chocolate milk; cream; ice cream, milk sherbets, whole-milk yogurt
Meat group	
Meats—6 ounces of skinned chicken or turkey, cod, haddock, halibut, clams, crab, lobster, oysters, scallops, perch, water-packed tuna or salmon; limit lean beef, veal, lamb, pork chops, and ham to 3 ounces three times per week	Fried meats; kidney, liver, brains, sweetbreads; shrimp, caviar, mackerel, any fish canned in oil; corned beef brisket, spareribs, pork butt, sausage, luncheon meats, frankfurters, bacon; duck, goose
Cheese—fat-free cottage cheese or sapsago	All other cheeses, including cream cheese
Eggs—egg substitutes or egg whites	Egg yolks
Fruit group	
All fruits and juices; avocado may be used in small amounts	None
Vegetable group	
All vegetables, including potatoes	None except those creamed or fried
Bread and cereal group	
All breads, plain rolls, English muffins, melba toast, rusks, crackers, pretzels, matzos; all cereals cooked or cold; spaghetti, macaroni; rice, hominy; baked goods and other products containing no whole milk or egg yolks and made with allowed fat	Hot breads, breads containing egg yolks; pancakes, doughnuts, sweet rolls, waffles, cheese crackers and other flavored crackers, potato chips, corn chips, egg noodles; commercial mixes; all tortillas

*The patient would also do well to write for Diet 2 for hypercholesterolemia, DHEW Publication No. (NIH) 74-112.

| **Foods permitted** | **Foods to avoid** |

Miscellaneous

| Seasonings—all spices and flavorings | None |

Fats—3 teaspoons of margarine such as Fleischmann's, Mazola, Saffola, Chiffon; 3 tablespoons of vegetable oil such as corn oil, cotton seed oil, safflower; French dressing or other oil dressings made from the above oils; nuts, nonhydrogenated peanut butter; olives

Olive oil, coconut oil; bacon fat, lard, hydrogenated fats, butter; gravies, cream sauces; cashews, macadamia nuts

Soups—fat-free broths and consommé, soups made with skim milk

All soups made with whole milk or cream; meat broths or bases with fat

Desserts and sweets—fresh and canned fruits; gelatin desserts, meringues, cornstarch puddings, rennet desserts made with skim milk; angel food cake, arrowroot cookies; fruit ices and whips made with egg whites, water sherbets; frosting without fat; sugar, honey, jelly, jams, syrups, hard candies, marshmallows, gumdrops

All others, including desserts, sweets, and candies containing chocolate or coconut

Beverages—coffee (regular or decaffeinated), tea, fruit juices, carbonated beverages, cocoa

None except chocolate

LOW-CHOLESTEROL SAMPLE MENU

All foods are cooked without added fat. Fat is trimmed off all meat.

Breakfast	**Dinner**	**Supper**
½ cup frozen orange juice	2 ounce tuna patty with lemon slice	3 ounces baked chicken (no skin)
½ cup oatmeal	1 medium baked potato	½ cup rice
1 low-cholesterol egg (example: Eggbeaters)	½ cup gingered banana squash	½ cup broccoli with lemon slice
1 slice toast	1 cup tossed salad	½ medium sliced tomato on leaf lettuce
1 teaspoon margarine	2 tablespoons corn oil with vinegar dressing	1 tablespoon corn oil with vinegar dressing
1 tablespoon jelly	2 peach halves in syrup	½ cup applesauce
1 cup skim milk	1 slice bread	1 slice bread
2 teaspoons sugar	1 teaspoon margarine	1 teaspoon margarine
coffee or tea	1 cup skim milk	1 cup skim milk
	1 teaspoon sugar	1 teaspoon sugar
	coffee or tea	coffee or tea

Prevention of endocarditis

Endocarditis, complicating valvular lesions or congenital heart abnormalities, is prevented by giving an antibiotic before, during, and for three days after any procedure that will predictably release bacteria into the bloodstream.

    I. Who should have prophylaxis?
       A. Patients with documented valvular disease, rheumatic or otherwise, of any variety.
       B. Congenital heart lesions, with rare exceptions. (Ask your physician about this.)
   II. What is the method of prophylaxis?*
       A. For all dental procedures or any surgical manipulations of the upper respiratory tract
          1. Penicillin G, one million units, procaine penicillin 600,000 units, intramuscular 30 to 60 minutes before procedure.
             Penicillin V, 500 milligrams by mouth every 6 hours for 8 doses. (Smaller doses are used for children.)
          2. Penicillin V, 2 grams by mouth 30 to 60 minutes before the procedure; 500 milligrams penicillin V every 6 hours for 8 doses thereafter.
          3. Alternative: Same doses of penicillins as listed above with 1 gram of streptomycin intramuscularly after surgery.
          4. For patients allergic to penicillin—one gram of vancomycin intravenously 30 to 60 minutes before procedure, 500 milligrams erythromycin by mouth every 6 hours for 8 doses.
       B. For surgical procedure or instrumentation of the genitourinary or gastrointestinal tracts
          1. Penicillin G, 2 million units or 1 gram of ampicillin, plus gentamicin intramuscularly or intravenously prior to procedure. Gentamicin plus penicillin or ampicillin every 8 hours for 2 doses after surgery.
          2. Streptomycin, 1 gram 30 to 60 minutes prior to procedure, the same dose together with penicillin every 12 hours for 2 doses after the procedure. (Smaller doses for children.)
       C. Prophylaxis in pregnancy
          1. It should be emphasized that pregnancy constitutes an invasion of the genitourinary tract with frequent release of bacteria into the bloodstream; patients with heart disease of the types listed above must have prophylaxis for endocarditis at the time of delivery.
          2. Recommendation: Procaine penicillin, 1.2 million units plus 1 gram streptomycin intramuscularly at the time of the onset of labor. Prophylaxis should be continued for three days after delivery.

---

*Recommendations of the American Heart Association.